Ready, Set, Eat!
Gluten-Free Nutrition Basics

A User-Friendly Guide to Gluten-, Casein-, Yeast-, and Allergen-free
Nutrition with Dietary Programs and Recipes for Individuals with Celiac Disease,
Gluten Sensitivity, ADD, ADHD, and Autism Spectrum Disorders

Faye Elahi, MS, MA
Gluten Sensitive Nutritionist

Ready, Set, Eat!
Gluten-Free Nutrition Basics

A User-Friendly Guide to Gluten-, Casein-, Yeast-, and Allergen-free Nutrition with Dietary Programs and Recipes for Individuals with Celiac Disease, Gluten Sensitivity, ADD, ADHD, and Autism Spectrum Disorders

Published by Nutrition Balance for Life, LLC

Copyright © 2011 by Faye Elahi
12880 Hillcrest Drive, Suite 105
Dallas, Texas 75230

Photography © by Dick Patrik/Dick Patrik Studios
Photography page 56: Orange © by Mike Rutherford; Cookie © Stockbyte®
CD5/Food Cutouts 2; Chips and Pretzels © Stockbyte® CD3/Food Cutouts 1

This cookbook is a collection of favorite recipes, which are not necessarily original recipes.

ISBN: 978-0-615-38312-5

Edited, Designed, and Produced by

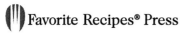 Favorite Recipes® Press

An imprint of

A wholly owned subsidary of Southwestern/Great American, Inc.
P. O. Box 305142
Nashville, Tennessee 37230
1-800-358-0560

Art Director and Book Design: Starletta Polster
Project Manager: Cathy Ropp
Recipe Editor: Georgia Brazil

Manufactured in the United States of America
First Printing: 2011
4,000 copies

Table of Contents

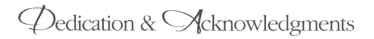

Dedication & Acknowledgments

To my mother and late father whose encouragements
have made me the person that I am
and to all the special parents whose passion is to unconditionally
love and serve their children.

Faye Elahi, MS, MA

I am grateful to the many people who have been instrumental in the production of this book. My husband and children have provided me the emotional support and understanding necessary for this book to become a reality.

Lynn Cook has been a devoted assistant whose support has been invaluable. At the initial phases of this book, Robyn Short contributed to getting this project started.

My medical partners have inspired me with their wisdom. The best diagnostician I have ever known, the late William Merritt Jr., MD, has left a legacy to treat the whole person using nutrition as an adjunct to medicine. I often think of his humanitarian soul. I thank Margaret Christensen, MD, for her loving energy and vision of total health. I am grateful to a forward-thinking gastroenterologist, Kenneth Fine, MD, who continues to offer a series of innovative stool tests that have been useful to my clients.

Renee Rossi, MD, mother of two, another intuitive physician, generously offered her time to review the manuscript in addition to sharing her wisdom as a mother and an otolaryngologist. I am especially grateful for her willingness to invest countless hours on this project, for believing in my preventive approach to health management, and for sharing her thoughts in the foreword of this book.

I also thank Alex Bekker, MD, homeopathic medicine physician, for treating many of my clients along with other physicians who believed in my integrative nutrition approach.

Last but not least, I owe my insight and clinical data to the thousands of my clients whose patience and commitment to finding a cure for themselves and their children is humbling. They are my heroes who grasp the meaning of selflessness.

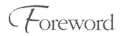

Faye Elahi brings her many years of clinical and personal experience along with sound scientific data to this user-friendly book on nutrition for those affected with celiac disease, attention deficit disorder, and autism spectrum disorders. In addition to providing sound advice on nutrition, Faye provides a number of recipes for delicious meals that are gluten-free and low in sugar. But this book does not stop there: it offers a nutritional foundation program for all people who wish to be healthy. We all remember the adage, "You are what you eat." In this day and age, many of us are not sure what we're eating, and we certainly have no idea what toxins and chemicals enter our bodies through our food, water, air, and environment. Though we cannot control certain toxins that are now ubiquitous in our environment, we can certainly decrease or limit our toxic burden by paying attention to exactly what we ingest.

Years ago, I met Faye while I was embarking on a detoxification program. I was experiencing increasing symptoms from inhalant allergies and was taking nasal steroids, antihistamines, and decongestants in increasing doses. I also had problems with chronic yeast infections, eczema, and gastroesophageal reflux (heartburn). As a physician, I suspected I might have some type of intestinal dysbiosis; however, I was treated with antireflux medications, frequent doses of oral antifungal medications, allergy medications, and topical steroids. It seemed as if I would never be able to discontinue these medications. Stool testing revealed I was gluten- and casein-sensitive. I went through an elimination diet and a cleanse and re-introduced foods one by one, confirming the gluten and casein sensitivities. In addition, I started on a low-sugar diet, multivitamins with minerals, probiotics, and fish oil. Within one year, I was off all my medications and only infrequently now have a mild outbreak of eczema. As of publication, I have been off all medications for eight years and have more energy! All of this makes intuitive sense as well. For many years, I would notice increasing allergy symptoms in my adult ENT practice, and it never made sense to me that allergies would increase as one grew older. Indeed, the toxic burden increases as one grows older, and the body's reaction to these toxins stimulates the immune system. Though we have many wonderful "band-aids" with modern medicine, we do not want to become pharmacologic cripples. I believe that anything we can do to take charge of our health will only improve the quality of our lives.

Thus, I am a convert and a believer in Faye's Nutrition Foundation Program for all people. As a physician, I truly believe we are working optimally when we act as facilitators for people to take the onus of responsibility for their own health to the degree they can. Faye Elahi provides us a toolbox in this excellent, life-affirming book.

Renee Rossi, MD

Dr. Rossi trained in Otolaryngology (ENT) at Ohio State University Hospitals and worked as faculty member at Harvard Medical School for seven years in the 90s. Dr. Rossi is currently a Clinical Assistant Professor in Otolaryngology at University of Texas Southwestern Medical School.

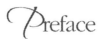
Preface

The purpose of this book is to present the latest and most effective nutritional and dietary programs that can be used as a general guide for individuals to optimize health. The guidelines are based on results seen in clients affected by attention deficit disorder, hyperactivity disorder, celiac disease, and gluten sensitivity, as well as autism spectrum disorders. The cases discussed consist of real people with modified names to protect their privacy, and the information is based on clinical progress notes, biomedical test results, and clients' reports.

Much of science is predicated on observation and data collection. During the past 20 years, I have observed the effects of diet and environmental inputs on health and have collected data; that is the basis of *my Nutrition Foundation Program.*

In Part I: The User Guide, I address *what we need to know* about our Western diet, the toxins that surround us, and their combined effects on our health. At the end, I offer step-by-step techniques that have helped my clients manage challenging diets free of gluten, casein, lactose, yeast, and food allergens with tips on how to feed a picky eater.

Part II: The Recipe Guide is an easy-to-follow cookbook which puts it all together in a 4-week menu as well as full-color pictures of about 20 of the most popular menu items. These mouthwatering dishes should motivate anyone to start on the *Nutrition Foundation Program.*

As a mother of two children with food allergies, I have shared my story to hopefully inspire other mothers or individuals to take charge of their health. To read my complete story, visit my Web site at *www.glutenfreenutritionforlife.com.* Enjoy!

Disclaimer—*This book is not intended to diagnose, treat, or cure any disease. Consult with a licensed physician for individualized treatment plans to manage your health.*

My Mission of Nutrition ...

Growing up, I was a thin, slightly anemic girl (low blood iron level) with chronic headaches. In my teens, while away from home, I discovered carbohydrate-rich foods. Gradually, I stopped menstruating (amenorrhea), developed chronic fatigue, and had difficulty retaining information. Subsequently, I reduced the starchy carbohydrates and revamped my diet in favor of organic vegetables and fruits. However, despite all these positive changes, I continued to have headaches, lack of retention, and anemia! It was health, not vanity, that prompted my quest for a specific diagnosis.

This journey spread over the next 18 years and included several sophisticated blood tests and endoscopies (an endoscopy consists of a tube inserted by a gastroenterologist into the small intestine to take cell samples). By 30, I had developed restless leg and slight peripheral neuropathy (numbness at the fingertips and toes). Finally my search for the truth led me to a Dallas gastroenterologist who diagnosed me with gluten sensitivity! At last, I had a valid scientific diagnosis which explained all my physical and psychological symptoms such as anxiety, irritability, foggy brain, chronic headache (ataxia), anemia, hypothyroidism, restless leg, peripheral neuropathy, and osteoporosis!

Like every newly diagnosed patient, I experienced the following gamet of emotions—denial, anger, and acceptance—only to realize that both patients and doctors have to become more aware of the *silent signs of celiac disease* or *gluten sensitivity.* Doctors should start screening high-risk individuals from European descent, like myself, or those with auto-immune diseases (Type I diabetes) for celiac disease and or gluten sensitivity. These people's desperate search for the right diagnosis is costing the American health care billions of unnecessary dollars when a simple genetic test could screen them and possibly save their lives!

Faye Elahi, MS, MA

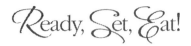

Part I: The User Guide

Why Do We Need the Nutrition Foundation Program (NFP)?

The Nutrition Foundation Program (NFP) is a core nutrition program that has been designed and used with great success on over 1,000 of my clients to optimize their health. The NFP is effective in managing everyone's nutritional health, especially those with

1. Celiac disease and gluten sensitivity
2. Attention deficit disorder with or without hyperactivity
3. Autism spectrum disorders

The Nutrition Foundation Program

- identifies nutritional deficiencies early on and designs dietary changes or nutrient supplementation to restore those deficiencies.
- increases each person's success rate by customizing the diet and supplements.
- simplifies steps in order to increase compliance to diet and supplements.
- is a scientific approach as all interventions are evidence based.
- is third party reimbursed in some states.

Genetic Predispositions

Each individual comes into the world with unique genetic coding that predisposes him or her to particular tendencies towards health as well as illness. Although our genetics do predispose us to a defined set of wellness possibilities, we are not necessarily doomed for illness nor destined for health. Genetic predispositions are greatly influenced by our environmental inputs as well as our nutritional intake. If we are predisposed to a particular illness and live mindlessly in a toxic environment, eating foods with "mysterious synthetic ingredients" and no vitamins to support our stressed bodies, the illness has a better chance of manifestation. However, the opposite is also true. If an individual has a predisposition to a certain illness but maintains a healthy environment with optimal nutrition, the illness or disorder may not manifest itself; or perhaps it will manifest in its mildest state.

Celiac disease, non-celiac gluten sensitivity, autistic spectrum disorder (ASD), pervasive developmental disorder (PDD), as well as attention deficit disorder

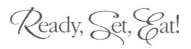

(ADD), and attention deficit hyperactivity disorder (ADHD) result from genetic predispositions triggered by a combination of environmental, psychological, and/or dietary inputs that provide the right circumstances for the particular conditions to manifest themselves.

Your Body Is a Temple

Most people have heard the expression, "Your body is a temple." A temple is the dwelling place for that which is sacred and important. The foods we eat and drink are the foundation of our body's health. A nutrient-dense diet provides a *solid foundation* for the temple, while a diet that contains synthetic foods lacking in vitamins and minerals will create a *shaky foundation* that will not maintain health. The environment in which a person lives, paired with his or her particular lifestyle, comprises the supporting structures of the temple—the framing, walls, and roof. The topography of the temple is its genetic makeup. The genetic makeup is important to the individual, such as those with a chromosomal abnormality which could cause developmental delays. Whether inherited or a *de novo* event, a genetic abnormality cannot always be predicted; however, migration studies show that genetic predispositions are linked, for the most part, to lifestyle factors like smoking, alcohol consumption, exercise, and nutrition. Nutrition is the one sure factor we can fully control most of the time that greatly influences our health. Can we eat perfectly 100 percent of the time? No! But searching for and selecting the right nutrients most of the time at the supermarket, farmers' market, and restaurant is possible.

What Is Your Body's Toxic Burden?

Everyone is born with a body toxic burden stemming from exposure to chemicals contained in drinking water, air, pesticides, processed foods, and pharmaceutical drugs, the sum of which delivers a significant toxic punch to a newborn.

The case of prebirth toxicity is illustrated by one of my four-year-old clients, Ben, a sweet boy diagnosed at age three with encephalopathy manifested by pervasive developmental disorder and autism spectrum disorder. His mother was diagnosed with severe hyperemesis gravidarum (HG), or extreme morning sickness. This led to her being prescribed a strong antinausea drug which, coupled with a delivery inducing drug, added up to a significant body toxic

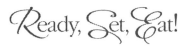

burden in both mother and infant. For a detailed account of Ben's case, please refer to his case study on page 40.

Other cases involve exposure to various toxins after birth. Toxins are in the food we eat and in the food our food eats (i.e. cattle feed, chicken feed, etc.). We absorb toxins through carpet, paint, household cleaners, and detergents. Many harmful organic components, such as xenoestrogens, are not screened by water filtration systems. Xenoestrogens are estrogen mimickers that act like estrogen in our bodies.

For the sake of our discussion, we will focus on the following foods that are found in a typical pantry or refrigerator, and, if ingested frequently, can add to a body's toxic burden: pesticide-contaminated produce, growth hormones and antibiotics in milk, artificial additives, preservatives, trans fats, and high fructose corn syrup.

Sodium Nitrite/Nitrate

These preservatives are used mostly in the meat industry to maintain color and freshness. Center for Science in the Public Interest (CSPI) has reported associations between these preservatives and the formation of small amounts of nitrosamines (cancer-causing chemicals). Fortunately, you can purchase several brands of deli meats or fresh meats that are free of these preservatives at your health food stores or local organic farms (see Shopping Guide on page 134). *Source:* The Green Guide, January/February 2006

Artificial Colors

Most of these colorings such as Blue #1, Blue #2, Green #3, Red # 3, and Yellow #6 have been tested by the CSPI and considered "most risky." Many of these are possibly linked to cancers and some to hyperactivity in children. If the word "lake" is used on the label such as "Blue Lake #3," that coloring contains aluminum, which is a toxic metal that everyone, especially young children, should minimize their exposure to.

High Fructose Corn Syrup (HFCS)

This is a genetically modified form of a corn derivative. Among the side effects are magnesium imbalance associated with osteoporosis; fatty acid increase linked

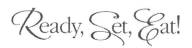
to heart disease; and higher risk of Type II diabetes. Many recent studies have linked higher use of HFCS to the rise in obesity, which stands at about 40 percent of the U.S. population.

Aspartame, Saccharine, and Acesulfame Potassium

Aspartame, known as NutraSweet, Equal, and Spoonful, has been associated with 75 percent of the negative side effects to food additives reported to the Food and Drug Administration (FDA). For a full listing of the negative side effects of aspartame, read Dr. Janet Hull's well researched book, *Sweet Poison*. Unlike saccharine that is not absorbed by humans, aspartame is digested and deposited in our tissues. Acesulfame potassium, which is commonly used in sweetening hand-scooped yogurts, has been reportedly linked to certain forms of cancer in rats.

Trans Fats or Hydrogenated Fats

Trans fats, also called hydrogenated or partially hydrogenated oils, are fake fats. The hydrogenated fats were made solid by adding a hydrogen atom in the wrong place. America loved them for their long shelf life and for their butter-like functionality. "It is like making plastic," according to Dr. Brain Olshansky, MD, a cardiologist and University of Iowa health care professor of internal medicine. He recommends that we minimize our trans fats because, as he warns, "Your body can't break them down." Because trans fats are stiff fats, Dr. Olshansky links them to obesity, heart disease, diabetes, high cholesterol, and even sudden cardiac death! It is noteworthy that some sources of trans fats such as unwrapped donuts, cookies, French fries, chips, and other *unlabeled products* can pass under the government labeling radar, as the 2006 labeling laws apply only to packaged foods! For instance, according to a study conducted by researchers at Gentofte University Hospital in Denmark and published in the New England Journal of Medicine, a large meal of chicken nuggets and French fries at McDonald's in the United States contained 10.1 grams of trans fatty acids; interestingly, the same meal contained 5.9 grams in France and just 0.33 grams in Denmark, Steen Stender, research project leader, told Agency of the French Press (AFP). This study startled me with its findings that a large meal of chicken nuggets and French fries from McDonald's contained nine times more unhealthy fats in the U.S. than in Denmark!

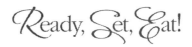

It Is a Toxic Environment!

The physical health of a nation of people is directly related to the health of
its soil. Over the course of the last 80 years, America's soil has become
increasingly less healthy. With the decline of our nation's soil, our waterways,
and our air, the food we eat has consequently become less healthy. The result is
obvious: we, as individuals, are less healthy than Americans who lived in the
early decades of the twentieth century.

A review of research published by the Unites States Department of Agriculture
(USDA) Data Laboratory shows that over the past two decades, calcium in the soil
has declined by an estimated 50 percent; magnesium has declined by 5 percent;
and potassium declined by as much as 30 percent. According to the editor of *Ode*
magazine, Marco Vissher, since 1985 the vitamin and mineral content of beans
has fallen by 60 percent, potatoes by 70 percent, and apples by 80 percent. Mass
farming practices, single crop farming known as monoculture, chemical pesticides
and fertilizers paired with Genetically Modified Organism (GMO) farming
practices, and GMO seeding have all pillaged the soil of its natural resources.
The trickle-down effects of polluted soil are polluted waterways and air, along
with pesticide- and petroleum-sprayed fruits and vegetables we consume. We
are even using arsenic in chicken diets to stimulate their appetite, or dichloro-
diphenyl-trichloroethane (DDT) in produce to feed cattle. The following diagram
is an oversimplified illustration of the lifecycle of toxic chemicals.

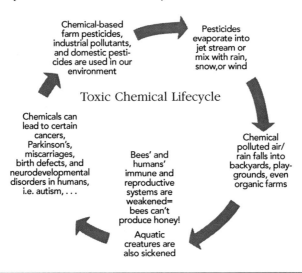

Toxic Chemical Lifecycle

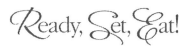
In recent years, regular milk, a common staple in everyone's diet, has become a common food allergen. In my clinic, about 70 percent of the children walk in with a severe or moderate milk allergy! In my adult population, this rate drops to about 50 percent perhaps due to children's high consumption of milk and cheese. It is a fact that the raw milk advocates have encouraged drinking milk from cows being fed natural green grass. However, most modern milk comes from cows fed a disproportionate amount of grains, and the milk is pasteurized and homogenized. Homogenization is a process whereby all the fat molecules are mechanically forced to be the same size so the cream is dispersed throughout. Currently the evidence is mounting against the use of homogenization. One such evidence is that the original fat molecule's membrane is broken, and a new one is formed that incorporates much larger amount of casein and whey proteins, potentially leading to milk-related allergies. The other evidence is related to the type of A1 beta-casein, mostly from Holstein cows, which is linked to "opiate-like" reaction in children with autism. According to Professor Boyd Swinburn's 2004 report to the New Zealand Food Safety Authority, "A1 beta-casein from cow's milk might cause or aggravate Type I diabetes, heart disease, schizophrenia, and autism." Although Professor Swinburn suggests that individuals at risk for developing these diseases reduce or remove the A1 beta-casein, he agrees that the benefits of this approach are unknown. For a more in-depth study of the A2 beta-casein, I suggest that you read *Devil in the Milk* by Keith Woodford.

In short, we have indirectly created this toxic environment—a depleted soil, producing depleted foods which have created depleted people! We can change it by going back to a self-sustaining farming style that supports the people as well as the globe.

A Nation of Overfed, Undernourished, and Underactive People

In late sixties and seventies, a small group of doctors and health care professionals specializing in behavioral research offered a link between a processed food diet and a rise in crime, schizophrenia, hyperactivity, learning differences, and other emotional disorders. Barbara Reed Stitt, a former chief probation officer from Ohio, has been a fervent advocate of controlling "junk food" as a significant method of reducing behaviors associated with "criminal behavior." In her book *Food and Behavior,* she notes that providing criminals, or anyone else, a diet rich

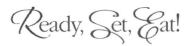

in whole grain breads, fruits, vegetables, and protein improved their behavior, attitude, and appearance dramatically.

The standard American diet is high in bad fats: saturated fats and trans fats, which are disease-causing fats deficient in essential fatty acids, omega 3, and 9 fatty acids.

In short, the American diet is overly sweet and loaded with starchy carbohydrates (pizza, bagels, pasta, bread) and unhealthy fats (fried food, ice cream). My internal study of over 1,000 families' diets showed a scary average sugar intake of 122 grams, or 24 teaspoons, of sugar a day! Unfortunately sugar from cereals, pastas, snacks, etc., can make up to 60 percent of the children's total diet! A 3-year-old was having as much as 20 teaspoons of sugar daily, disguised as fruit juice, yogurt, low-fat desserts, and snacks. Fast foods are also more prevalent in our society than ever before because they are convenient and cheaper than healthy foods. The food industry pushes us to eat more with messages like "bigger is better!" Ads geared to children who have fewer natural cognitive defenses also drive them to eat more. All these factors along with our sedentary lifestyles have made us a **nation of overfed, undernourished, and underactive people.**

Laying the Nutrition Foundation: 6 Steps for the Whole Family

1. Limit the daily sugar intake to 30 grams (6 teaspoons) for children and 40 grams (8 teaspoons) for adults.
2. Reduce fast food intake from daily to occasionally.
3. Eliminate food allergens and excitotoxins (phenols in artificial colors and flavors).
4. Add high-quality multivitamin/mineral supplements (best if customized).
5. Add a high-quality probiotic.
6. Add a high-quality fish oil.

This core Nutrition Foundation Program is a base program for all people, with additional supplements for those with celiac disease, autism, and attention deficit hyperactivity disorder.

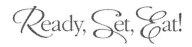
Step 1: Limit the daily sugar intake to 30 grams (6 teaspoons) for children and 40 grams (8 teaspoons) for adults.

This fits in with the American Diabetic Association recommendations for sugar intake. Other than the obvious sugar spike and agitation that simple sugar causes, followed by a sugar low, high amounts of simple sugar from processed foods like juices, desserts, candies, snacks, and cereals can slow bowel transit. This can increase the exposure of toxins to gut cell lining (mucosa). Here are some favorite family foods and their sugar content:

Food item	Sugar content
All-natural lemonade or orange juice	28 grams per cup (about 5 teaspoons)
Regular ketchup	9 grams per tablespoon/1 packet (2 teaspoons)
Girl Scout cookies	7 grams per 2 cookies (1.5 teaspoons)
Gummy bears	34 grams per 15 gummies (10 teaspoons)
Sugar-coated donut	65 grams (13 teaspoons)
Average can of soda	38 grams per 8 fluid ounces (about 8 teaspoons)
Popular children cereals	12–16 grams per 3/4 cup (2.5–3 teaspoons)

Interestingly, my pediatric and young adolescent populations do well when I use a simple tool to educate them about the negative effects of sugar: label reading! The most recent success story came from a group of 12-year-old girls wanting to lose about 10 pounds to improve their health. After tallying their dietary sugar intake, we found that they each were consuming more than 100 grams of sugar a day just from snacks! At my label reading session, they each were given the challenge of getting their sugar at or below 30 grams a day without increasing their activity (they were already enrolled in a daily 2-hour dance class). The average weight loss over two months was ten pounds per person! All of the girls told me that although at first it was challenging to stay within 30 grams of sugar a day, later it got easier. The parents tell me that these girls are still label readers even though they have reached their desired weight goals. The girls are satisfied with the lifestyle change because they feel empowered with the knowledge of

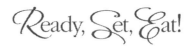

nutrition. I am sure that we have taught these girls how to prevent obesity by label reading and portion control. My mission of nutrition continues on.

Step 2: *Reduce fast food intake from daily to occasionally.*

There is no doubt that our fast food environment is toxic for susceptible people who regularly eat fast foods; their high content of trans fats, high fructose corn syrup, gluten, dairy, and multiple chemical preservatives is associated with chronic diseases like obesity and Type II diabetes. So if we want to change our health, we need to change the type of fast food consumption to include more vegetables and grilled lean chicken.

Step 3. *Eliminate food allergens and excitotoxins (phenols in artificial colors and flavors)*

I always recommend IgE (immediate–onset allergy reaction) as well as IgG (delayed-onset allergy reaction) tests to be done before I restrict someone's diet. Consequently, we always see noticeable improvements in behaviors and physical characteristics (eczema, rash, dark circles under eyes, etc.) after the problem foods are eliminated. The most common food allergens are: wheat, milk, eggs, peanuts, corn, and soybeans.

After the elimination period, we usually challenge the person to see if it is safe to reintroduce that food into the diet. A fail-proof method to discover a food reaction is by having a planned session where the old food allergen is eaten and symptoms monitored over three days. If no negative symptom manifests itself, the person can eat the food again, but on a four-day rotation basis to prevent the old food reactions.

Excitotoxins, or phenols, are found in artificial food additives commonly used in the processed food manufacturing industry to enhance both the flavor and texture of food. Glutamate, as monosodium glutamate (MSG), is a common flavor enhancer. This food additive overstimulates the nervous system and may damage brain cells, cause hyperactivity, high anxiety, and neurological dysfunction in some sensory hypersensitive people. Excitotoxins are linked to adult diseases such as Parkinson's, amyotrophic lateral sclerosis (ALS), Huntington's disease, Alzheimer's disease, and developmental and behavioral disorders in children. To do damage control in this area, it is prudent to avoid the following: monosodium

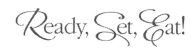

glutamate (MSG), hydrolyzed vegetable protein (HVP), hydrolyzed protein (HP), hydrolyzed plant protein (HPP), sodium caseinate, calcium caseinate, yeast extract, and autolyzed yeast. Phenols are also found in fake colorings.

Step 4: *Add high-quality multivitamin/mineral supplements.*
Adding high-quality multivitamin/mineral supplements is essential to building a strong nutritional foundation. Vitamins and minerals are noncaloric sources of nutrients that play a crucial role in facilitating the transport and absorption of food.

In my practice I am asked on a daily basis: "Can't my child get all of the nutrients he needs from food?" The answer is yes, IF your child gets sufficient nutrients from food. For example, in order to obtain enough vitamin D, a crucial vitamin for bone development and immune strength, a person would need to drink forty 8-ounce glasses of milk per day, eat three pounds of liver per day, or two pounds of fatty fish per day!

A "high-quality" multivitamin is one that is developed based on Good Manufacturing Practices (GMP) as defined by the U.S. Food and Drug Administration and free of the common food allergens: corn, wheat/gluten, soy, yeast, milk/dairy, sugar, salt, nuts, artificial colors and flavors, preservatives, pesticides, PCBs, toxic metals, and excipients. In many cases, due to multiple clinical challenges a child with celiac disease or autism is faced with, therapeutic-grade supplements are needed which are available through nutrition professionals and health care practitioners. However, the best nutritional supplements are those that are customized to meet the person's unique deficiencies as determined by urine or blood tests. In my practice, I follow a three-step program to customize multivitamins/minerals:

A. A comprehensive nutrition assessment is done to establish the person's baseline for nutrition and vitamin deficiencies as well as digestive health. This is done through either the primary physician, or a pediatrician associated with a trained nutritionist testing for 45 biomedical markers in a simple urine organic acid test.

B. Tests results are reviewed by the trained nutritionist and a medical doctor who can design a customized multivitamin formula to meet the person's unique deficiencies.

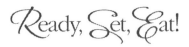

C. The customized multivitamin supplement program is combined with needed dietary eliminations and additions and other needed therapies (occupational, speech, music therapy, or applied behavior analysis therapies) to maximize benefits.

Step 5. *Add a high-quality probiotic.*

Probiotic means "for life." Probiotics are friendly living microorganisms, or "healthy microflora," that need to be taken in sufficient amounts to support gastrointestinal health. Since the gastrointestinal tract is host to trillions of bacteria, from 500 different varieties (more than cells in our body), alcohol consumption, antibiotics, spoiled foods, and exposure to toxic substances reduce friendly bacteria and shift the balance in favor of bad bacteria. This is the main reason why antibiotics make us feel tired. I recommend using a specific probiotic designed to allow the beneficial action of the antibiotic while lowering its negative side effect of killing the friendly flora. In general, for every week of antibiotic use, a probiotic should be taken for three weeks.

Probiotics may benefit you by strengthening the immune system; assisting in synthesis of B vitamins; promoting colon health and bowel regularity; helping the absorption of some minerals such as calcium; preventing or relieving diarrhea and abdominal pain; naturally inhibiting the growth of pathogenic bacteria by increasing intestinal acidity, which can cause disease-causing bacteria such as *Helicobacter pylori* (*H. pylori*, a bacterium causing ulcers to grow); and improving digestion of lactose by supporting lactase enzyme production (found in raw milk). I also recommend the use of raw fermented foods or coconut kefir rich in probiotics (see Shopping Guide for brands, page 134).

A good quality probiotic must contain the following: several billions of live cultures, preferably nondairy, made with live cultured bacteria. To choose the ideal probiotic for you, consult your health care professional or visit *www.glutenfreenutritionforlife.com.*

Whole Coconut—The Natural Probiotic!

Another key natural antifungal (anti-yeast) fruit is whole coconut, especially young, organic coconut. Its juice can be fermented into coconut kefir (pronounced ke-fur), a fatty acid rich in lauric acid which is known to boost the immune

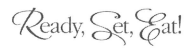

system. This fatty acid also has antifungal properties, so it is useful in yeast-free diets to combat yeast infections such as candidiasis. Until recently, the predominant scientific message was that coconut oil was a "saturated fat" or a bad fat! Research now shows that coconut oil's medium-chain fatty acids might help prevent chronic diseases. Specifically, lauric acid is a medium-chain fatty acid that is also found in breast milk and is known to boost the immune system. According to John Hopkins scientist Gerard Mullin, coconut oil promotes a good balance of LDL (bad cholesterol) and HDL (good cholesterol). Because of its fiber and protein contents, as well as its low digestible carbohydrates, I have used tasty coconut in many of my recipes in the later part of this book.

Step 6: *Add a high-quality fish oil.*

Good-quality fish oil should be derived from a wild fish source (not farm-raised). The content must be free of all the common allergens and should contain the important components of the DHA, EPA (omega-3 components in marine oils). Quality fish oils are free of detectable levels of mercury, lead, cadmium, and PCBs. I recommend contacting the manufacturer and requesting a statement of purity.

Children under the age of five should take a fish oil that is **higher in docosahexaenoic acid (DHA)** than eicosapentaenoic acid (EPA). DHA is a major building block of tissues in the brain and retina in the eye. DHA plays a role in forming neurotransmitters such as **phosphatidylserine**—a vital nutrient in normal nerve and brain function. Children above five and adults should take a fish oil supplement that is **higher in EPA** than DHA. EPA promotes healthy blood chemistry and prostaglandins, which regulate cell activity.

Fish oils play an important role in speech development and sensory processing among children with a deficit in this area. Children who have sensory processing disorder almost always benefit from fish oils by experiencing the following: improved mental clarity; decrease in emotional outbursts; decrease in transient mood; improved behavioral compliance; decreased irritability; increased calmness; improvement and/or elimination of "sideways glance;" and significant progress in speech, coordination, and motor planning. Fish oil must be given consistently at the right dosage for 90 days to lead to noticeable improvements.

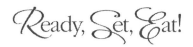

What is Candida and its connection with a Leaky Gut?

Candida is a type of pathogenic, or harmful, bacteria that grows in the gastrointestinal tract, which is a long hollow tube starting at the mouth and ending at the anus.

Candida, also known as yeast, can start at birth as the infant is born through the yeast-infected birth canal. Candida, or yeast overgrowth, can manifest itself as thrush, a vaginal yeast infection, a skin rash, itchy ears, or athlete's foot, or with emotional symptoms such as irritability, anxiety, restlessness, or even depression.

If the ratio of friendly bacteria, viruses, and fungi cohabitating in our digestive tract is tipped in favor of the pathogenic bacteria, the digestive tract cells are damaged, allowing the partially digested food particles to be absorbed into the bloodstream, causing a "leaky gut." Other factors can also damage the gut flora (bacteria colonies) such as infectious diseases, stress, sugary-starchy diet, antibiotic overuse, physical exertion, old age, alcoholism, pollution, exposure to toxins, and extreme climates. As a result of the leaky gut condition, the person often develops an overgrowth of yeast, or candida, which can cause many other health problems such as nutrient and vitamin malabsorptions. This in turn can lead to osteomalacia and rickets, also known as vitamin D deficiency; anemia or iron deficiency; folate deficiency; and pernicious anemia or vitamin B12 deficiency. These conditions are common among individuals diagnosed with autism, attention deficit disorder (hyperactivity disorder), celiac disease, gluten sensitivity, food allergies, dyspraxia, asthma, eczema, and learning differences. Apart from these childhood learning and neurological disorders, there is another group of conditions which are affected by the leaky gut. These conditions are bipolar disorder, obsessive compulsive disorder, depression, and schizophrenia. According to the father of French psychiatry Phillipe Pinel, (1745–1828): "The primary seat of insanity generally is in the region of the stomach and intestines."

Some biomedical signs of leaky gut are low or low/normal blood glucose, low serum calcium, low serum phosphate, high serum alkaline phosphatase, low serum albumin, and low serum potassium.

Possible underlying causes of a leaky gut
1. Hydrochloric Acid (HCL) insufficiency

This condition can be caused by abnormal gut flora (harmful bacteria) or overgrowth of pathogenic bacteria or candida, which can suppress stomach acid

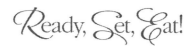

production. Since stomach acid allows digestive enzymes to do their job of breaking down large protein molecules into smaller pieces that are digestible, without sufficient acid production, the digestion of proteins becomes problematic. So, when a person has few friendly bacteria to protect the gut lining, toxins penetrate the gut wall and "leak" into the bloodstream, ending up in the brain, thus causing mental symptoms such as foggy brain or inattention or even speech impairement. The signs of low HCL production are:

- Bloating or belching immediately after meals
- Fullness after eating
- Itching around the rectum
- Weak, peeling, or cracked fingernails
- Post-adolescent acne
- Undigested food in stool

2. Pancreatic Enzyme insufficiency

An insufficiency of stomach hydrochloric acid can lead to low levels of pancreatic enzymes. Furthermore, candida can convert the sugar from our starchy foods into alcohol. The alcohol byproduct of dietary sugar can directly damage the gut lining, causing nutrient malabsorption and lower pancreatic enzyme production. Consequently, digestion of fats and starches becomes a problem which can lead to abdominal pain, weight loss, fatty stool, glucose intolerance, malnutrition, vitamin deficiencies (most commonly vitamins A and B), pale or bulky stool, foul smelling stool, abdominal bloating, and excess gas, to name a few.

How Can We Repair the Leaky Gut?
Elimination Diet

Reportedly, the majority of people respond favorably to the elimination of the top eight food allergens: dairy, gluten, corn, soy, shellfish, peanut, sugar, and egg. The elimination diet is by far the most effective way we can stop further damage to the gastro-intestinal system. Of course, the long-term success of people with multiple food allergies depends on how thoroughly they eliminate the problem foods as well as how carefully they reintroduce them into the diet, with attention to immune and digestive system reactions.

Specific Carbohydrate Diet

This diet was originally developed by an American pediatrician named Dr. Haas who saw a relationship between disaccharides (sucrose, maltose, and lactose)

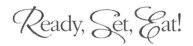

and intestinal damage. Although this diet is restrictive, it has been has been very helpful to some extreme celiacs and autistic individuals. (Refer to Elaine Gotschall's book *Breaking the Vicious Cycle*.)

Faye's Anti-Candida Diet

This diet rules out most breads as they call for yeast as the starter. My two-step anti-candida diet can be followed up to nine months to rid oneself of candida or yeast overgrowth.

Step I: 1 month (could be repeated)

Foods to Avoid	Foods Allowed
Sugar, Chocolate, Honey, Maltose, Maple Syrup, Sucrose	Stevia Sweetener, Dark Molasses Naturally Sweetened Coconut Juice, Coconut Products
Regular Fruit Juice, Dried Fruit	Unsweetened Cranberry Nectar (1/2 cup juice to 1/2 cup water) with Stevia
Apple, Grape, Mango, Banana, Watermelon	Pear, Grapefruit, Peach, Coconut
Baking Powder	Xanthan Gum (Gluten-Free Baking Leavening)
Yeast Breads, Grains (Rice, Wheat, etc.)	Quinoa, Amaranth
Regular Vinegar	Unsweetened Lemon Juice (fresh) with Stevia
Corn Products or High Fructose Corn Syrup	Agave Nectar
Beer, Alcohol, Sweet Drinks	Fresh Lime Juice or Green Tea with Stevia
Hard Candy, Dessert	Low Glycemic Index Bars, Coconut
Dairy, Moldy Cheeses (Cheddar, Blue)	Coconut Milk (contains caprilic acid: anti-yeast properties), Coconut Yogurt
White Potato, Corn	All Other Vegetables
Farm-raised Fish, Fat-tier Fish (such as Carp or Catfish due to possible high PCB content)	Meat, Chicken, Pork, Small Fish, Wild Salmon (antibiotic free)

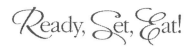

Step II: 3 months

Reintroduce a limited amount of dark chocolate (1 ounce); or half juice/half water combination (4 ounces); or any other of the avoided foods at the rate of one every four days to identify possible yeast symptoms. If symptoms reappear, repeat Steps I and II.

1. No soaking in a bubble bath during the anti-candida diet. This can invite yeast infections in the urinary tract or vaginal area.

2. Prepare the intestinal environment for good bacteria growth by drinking 1 tablespoon of apple cider vinegar mixed in 1 ounce water first thing upon rising while on the anti-candida diet or 1 ounce of young coconut kefir (see listing in Shopping Guide, page 134).*

3. Adding an herbal antimicrobial supplement containing agents such as sweet wormwood, caprilic acid, berberine sulfate, grapefruit seed extract, barberry, black walnut, and/or bearberry is recommended during Step I.

4. If amino acid deficiencies exist along with candida, first eliminate the candida, then add on the free-form amino acids.

5. If you should be averse to the taste of coconut kefir or apple cider vinegar, you may replace them with a broad spectrum, dairy- and gluten-free high-quality probiotic (minimum of 100-plus billion probiotic microorganisms per day).

6. Although antibiotics can save lives, in my experience they are not very effective in eradicating candida cases. The most effective way to eliminate candida or any other yeast/fungi is to "starve them out."

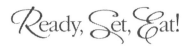

Feingold Diet

This diet is based on limiting a category of food that is rich in phenols and salicylates. All natural protein sources, fats, and carbohydrates contain phenols. Since 80 percent of all foods (including food coloring and popular fruits such as berries) need to be eliminated on this diet, most children find it too restrictive.

In a society where most children and adults have a leaky gut due to a combination of starchy diet, overexposure to prescription drugs, and a pool of toxic substances in the digestive tract, a simple dietary restriction is not going to cancel out the damage caused to the gut. What seems to reverse this damage is a combination of a low-sugar, anti-candida, and elimination diet to allow the lining of the gut to heal while adding a safe amount of high-quality probiotics to protect the gut wall from further damage by invading toxins. In most cases, we see remarkable improvements in behaviors of autistic and attention deficited individuals as the balance of friendly flora is restored and the diet is cleaned up.

How to Recognize Oral Motor Deficits

Typically a speech or feeding therapist is the right person to assess and diagnose oral motor deficits. Feeding issues can start at birth although most start at the time solid foods are introduced. In most children or adults with sensory processing deficits, the person typically gags or has projectile vomiting or they have picky eating habits. It is crucial to distinguish between the "problem eaters" and "picky eaters." Problem eaters usually end up with an aversion towards eating food versus picky eaters who eat but are very selective with the texture, taste, smell, and/or look of the foods they eat. For more on sensory processing disorder, read *The Out-of-Sync Child*, Carol Stock Kranowitz, MA.

The solution involves multiple steps as follows:
- Go back to the sensory age of the child and reintroduce soft favorite foods.
- Start eliminating one food group at a time (casein first, then gluten).
- Plan on stimulating the mouth with four tastes daily: salty (Lay's Stax Potato Chips), sour (tangerine, drops of lime juice), sweet (cookies), and bitter (gluten-free pretzels) daily. Keep a record of progress to report to team members like the nutritionist or feeding therapist (see sensory picture on page 49).

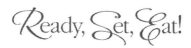

- Prepare for withdrawal symptoms (rise in maladaptive behaviors, low appetite).
- Physically stimulate the mouth with a therapeutic oral-motor device such as z-vibe (looks like a toothbrush with a rotating tip) based on the expert advice of a speech therapist.
- Start on customized multivitamins/minerals since a vitamin and mineral deficiency could be the main reason behind oral motor deficits!

How Do Oral Motor Deficits Affect Taste?

The deficiencies in certain minerals such as zinc and iron can affect the sense of taste in all of us. In general, when a person's mineral and vitamin deficiencies are corrected, the sense of taste improves, and consequently the person is more willing to try new foods.

Strategies to Get the Picky Eater to Eat!

The following strategies have proven to work for picky eaters in my practice:

- Offer one new food with two old foods three or four times a week.
- Administer no corporal punishment for lack of cooperation in feeding.
- Rule out sensory component (feeding history).
- Change the environment where new foods are introduced (formal dining, etc.).
- Lengthen the time the child sits at the table (use a timer or new chair).
- Make a picture schedule.
- Limit snacks and "grazing" between meals.
- Ensure zinc deficiency is corrected.
- Invite older siblings, friends, and/or neighbors to model good eating.
- Introduce foods without expectations to eat (play is fine).
- Vary the texture of foods from crunchy to soft and chewy to stimulate the muscles involved in chewing and swallowing.

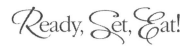

Nutrition Foundation Program (NFP) for Celiac Disease and Gluten Sensitivity

Understanding Celiac Disease

Up until the early 1990s, celiac disease was considered a rare condition in the United States and Europe when 1 in every 5,000 people were thought to have the disease. Today, according to the Mayo Clinic, 1 in every 100 people is believed to suffer from celiac disease (over 3 million in the U.S.). Celiac disease, also known as "celiac sprue," is an immune-mediated genetic disease in which gluten damages the small intestinal mucosa, or the intestinal lining. Gluten is the protein portion of wheat, barley, spelt, and rye, and only contaminated oats, millet, and sorghum. This serious genetically mediated disease could, if ignored, possibly lead to certain forms of cancer and eventually death.

Inversely, if one is diagnosed early and implements a gluten-free diet, one can correct the symptoms and lead a healthy life. Dr. Peter Green, Professor of Clinical Medicine for the College of Physicians and surgeons at Columbia University, studied 10 million subscribers to CIGNA and found those who were correctly diagnosed with celiac disease used fewer medical services and reduced their healthcare costs by 30 percent!

Signs and Symptoms of Celiac Disease

For a comprehensive listing of all 250 symptoms, read James Brady, MD's outstanding book, *Dangerous Grains*. These include the following: iron deficiency or iron deficiency anemia, folate and vitamin B12 deficiency, elevated serum alkaline phosphatase linked to bone loss, low serum albumin, abdominal distention (bloating), chronic or intermittent diarrhea or constipation, stunted growth, autism, alopecia (hair loss or thinning), osteoporosis (children with low-impact bone fractures), epilepsy (history of migraines), ADHD, major depression unresponsive to pharmaceuticals, itchy-blistering rash (dermatitis herpetiformis), early menopause, febrile seizures, gallstones, dental enamel defects, delayed puberty, muscular hypotonia (low muscle tone), neurological disorders, pica (eating non-foods like dirt, clay, etc.), and lupus erythematosus. If a person ignores the diagnosis of celiac, their risk of serious medical diseases such as cancer or autoimmune diseases like Sjögren's syndrome and rheumatoid arthritis can increase by up to 40 percent.

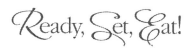

Non-Celiac Gluten Sensitivity

Gluten sensitivity is an umbrella diagnosis that may lead to other diagnoses including but not limited to celiac disease, dermatitis herpetiformis, Sjögren's syndrome, or gluten ataxia depending on genetic factors. According to many scientists, over 90 million Americans are affected by non-celiac gluten sensitivity. Gluten sensitivity is believed to be very common, and yet it is screened and diagnosed even less frequently than celiac disease. I was one of these hard-to-diagnose individuals who had a few typical and many atypical symptoms. Early diagnosis could prevent further development of other diseases.

What Parents of Celiac Children Need to Know

Celiac is a lifelong diagnosis. If a child tests positive for celiac disease, both parents should also be tested, as celiac is a genetic disease. Almost all my young celiac clients have grown in large measure within 6 to 12 months following the NFP for celiacs (see page 29). The following CELIAC acronym offers lifestyle guidelines for people with celiac and gluten sensitivity:

C – Consultation with a nutritionist who specializes in celiac disease and gluten sensitivity.

E – Education about the disease.

L – Lifelong adherence to a gluten-free diet.

I – Identification and treatment of nutritional deficiencies.

A – Access to an advocacy group.

C – Continuous long-term follow-up.

How Early Can I Test My Child for Celiac Disease?

According to Ivor D. Hill, MD, Professor of Pediatrics at Wake Forrest University School of Medicine, early onset of gastrointestinal symptoms typically occurs in children between 6 and 18 months of age unless the breastfeeding mother is eating gluten or the baby is exposed to shampoos, lotions, and other products containing gluten.

The chart on the following page simplifies your testing options with the pros and cons of each test.

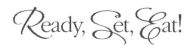

Test	Cost of Test	Positive	Negative
Upper GI Endoscopy	High	Gives definitive results	Invasive. Can cause a sore throat for 2–3 days and requires anesthesia
Blood Test: Anti-Tissue Transglutaminase IgG	Varies	Cost is relatively low if the individual has insurance.	Invasive (needle stick). Cannot prove gluten sensitivity due to partial damage to small bowel
Blood Test: Anti-Tissue Transglutaminase IgA	Varies	Cost is relatively low if the individual has insurance.	Invasive. Unreliable in cases of partial damage to the small bowel (false negative results)
Blood Test: Total IgA	Varies	Has a high reliability factor since it can pick up partial damage to the small intestine.	Cost: Insurance covers only about 20 percent in most cases
Blood Test: Endomysial Antibody IgA Reflex (if indicated by the results of positive Total IgA)	Varies	If your insurance plan pays for the test, cost is economical.	Cannot prove gluten sensitivity due to partial damage to small bowel
Blood Test: Anti-Gliadin IgA/IgG Add-on blood test	Varies	Can prove gluten sensitivity and celiac disease.	Cannot prove gluten sensitivity due to partial damage to small bowel
Stool Test: Gluten Sensitivity Stool test	approximate cost $125	Non-invasive procedure gives definitive results	Cannot confirm celiac disease

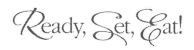

Vitamin Deficiencies of People with Celiac

Celiacs typically develop nutritional malabsorption due to damaged lining of the small intestine. As a result, the individual can develop a permeable or leaky gut. Commonly, celiacs report varying degrees of deficiencies including calcium (hypocalcaemia), magnesium, manganese, selenium, copper, iron (anemia), and zinc as well as vitamins A, most Bs, C, D, E, and K.

Nutrition Foundation Program (NFP) for Celiac Disease and Gluten Sensitivity

1. *Limit the daily sugar intake to 30 grams (6 teaspoons) for children and 40 grams (8 teaspoons) for adults.*
2. *Reduce fast food intake from daily to occasionally.*
3. *Eliminate food allergens and excitotoxins (phenols in artificial colors and flavors).*
4. *Add high-quality multivitamin/mineral supplements (best if customized).*
5. *Add a high-quality probiotic*
6. *Add a high-quality fish oil.*

In addition to the above six steps of NFP (explained starting on page 14), I recommend the following important add-ons:

7. *Eliminate gluten (grain protein).*
8. *Eliminate casein (dairy protein).*
9. *Add digestive enzymes.*
10. *Add amino acids as needed.*

Step 7. *Eliminate Gluten (grain protein).*

- **Foods Allowed on a Gluten-Free Diet:** Amaranth, Arrowroot, Bean Flours (Fava, Garfava, Garbanzo), Buckwheat (unless in a mix with gluten flours), Kasha (toasted Buckwheat), Corn (including Corn Bran, Cornmeal, Corn Grits, Hominy), Flax Seed (including Flaxseed Meal), Millet Seed, Montina Flour, Nut Flours, Potato Flour, Potato Starch, Tef, Quinoa Seed (including Quinoa Flour), Rice, Sorghum Flour, Soy Flour, and Tapioca.

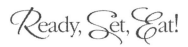

- **Foods to Avoid on a Gluten-Free Diet:** Barley (Malted Barley, Malt Extract, Malt Flavoring, Malt Syrup, Malt Vinegar), Bulgar, Couscous, Dinkel, Durum, Einkom, Farro, Graham Flour, Kamut, Oats (Oat Bran, Oat Syrup except certified gluten-free oats or steel cut oats), Rye, Semolina, Spelt, Triticale, Wheat (Wheat Bran, Wheat Germ, or Wheat Starch except gluten-free wheat germ oil).
- **Hidden Non-food Sources of Gluten:** Keratin shampoos, hair products, lotions, pharmaceuticals, toothpastes, pet foods, cleaning products, skin care, make-up, wax papers, soaps, and gum, to name a few.

If abdominal pain, diarrhea, or nausea persist after eliminating gluten, eliminate disaccharides for one month per *Specific Carbohydrate Diet*, SCD, by Elaine Gotschall (see Sources). Since some celiacs have a deficiency of carbohydrate digesting enzymes for disaccharides (rice, corn, potatoes, soy, sugar, chocolate, jam pectins, and baking powder), the SCD, based on monosaccharides (beans, legumes, nuts, seeds, vegetables, fruit, fresh fruit juices, meat, eggs, ghee, honey), is better tolerated. Monosaccharides do not require digestive enzymes for absorption.

Step 8. *Eliminate casein (dairy protein).*
If you continue to have persistent abdominal issues such as diarrhea, bloating, gas, constipation, or nausea, then a casein and lactose intolerance test is needed to rule out the presence of these intolerances before restricting the diet. Most celiacs have lactose intolerance due to deficiency of lactase enzyme interrupted by villi damage. Some gluten-, lactose-, casein-free milk substitutes are almond, hemp, and rice milks. Oat milk is not gluten-free unless specified, and it is not well tolerated by most celiacs.

Step 9. *Add digestive enzymes.*
Digestive enzymes are necessary in cases of gastrointestinal malabsorption when there is proven deficiency of protein enzymes such as proteases (peptizyde). I often recommend a specific chewable enzyme containing lipase (fat digestion), amylase (carbohydrate digestion), and protease (protein digestion) to offer immediate relief. For best results, one has to first take a comprehensive digestive stool analysis to identify the specific missing enzymes, as well as possible

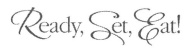

parasites or fungi, then treat with targeted digestive enzymes and antifungals, if necessary. If one does not see results by taking an over-the-counter enzyme, it may mean that it was not the right type of digestive enzyme for them.

Step 10. *Add amino acids as needed.*

Typically, most celiacs develop some form of malabsorption issue in the gut evidenced by a GI comprehensive stool analysis test. A serum amino acid deficiency test is usually ordered if clinical symptoms of such deficiencies are present such as lack of focus, agitation, or anxiety, to name a few.

Glutamine is an amino acid that the body produces when healthy. The benefits of it are elevated energy, concentration, and memory; healthy blood sugar; support for healthy muscle build-up for body builders; increased stress tolerance; and support of the entire gastrointestinal tract. Glutamine is often depleted in those with yeast overgrowth and is partly responsible for "brain fog." It is the primary energy source for the cells that line the intestines, and it keeps them healthy.

Case Studies

Marianne: 3-year-old girl

Diagnosed with celiac disease, Type II diabetes (adult onset diabetes), food allergies

Marianne was by Carol G. Kranowitz's definition, "an overresponsive child with sensory modulation problems" at age three. She had developed strong food aversions due to vitamin and mineral deficiencies, affecting her sense of taste at the source of her oral motor deficits. The more food aversions she had, the less variety of food she ate, and the more severe her vitamin and mineral deficiencies became. As she objected to foods, her parents gave in more to her wish to eat only starchy and sweet foods. This negatively reinforced her picky eating behaviors, eventually leading to Type II diabetes and celiac disease by age six.

She then started on the NFP and grew in weight and height and became less picky about foods in under one year. Today she is a happy girl who is on a gluten-free and diabetic diet.

(continued on next page)

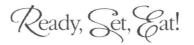

Marianne: 3-year-old girl

Before custom multivitamin/mineral supplements and NFP	After custom multivitamin/mineral supplements and NFP	Nutritional Supplements list
Short stature	Grew 3.4 inches in 3 months.	Combination of all the family of B Vitamins
Underweight	Gained 6 pounds in 3.5 months.	100-plus billion of broad spectrum dairy-free, gluten-free probiotic
Dental enamel defect Hypoglycemia Anemia B-12 and folate deficiencies Anorexia, malaise	Colors returned to normal. After 3 months on NFP, anemia corrected, inattention improved by about 50-60 percent per teachers.	Custom multivitamins and minerals
Nausea Headache Intermittent diarrhea	Nausea subsided. Headache eliminated when food allergies eliminated. Diarrhea stopped within days.	Extra zinc to restore sense of taste
Severe oral motor defensiveness and sensory integration deficits vitamin/mineral deficiencies	Daily encouragements aided in expanding diet to 12 foods; cut sugar to 30 grams per day.	Extra iron, selenium, and D vitamins

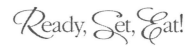

Daniel: 10-year-old boy

Diagnosed with gluten sensitivity, asthma, and food allergies

Before custom multivitamin/mineral supplements and NFP	After custom multivitamin/mineral supplements and NFP (gluten- and casein-free)	Nutritional Supplementation Program
Short stature	Grew 5 inches in 9 months.	Zinc to repair the epithelial cells of intestinal walls
Underweight	Gained 10 pounds in 9 months.	Minerals to heal the intestinal walls
Projectile vomiting	None after dairy elimination since milk caused inflammation and thickening of mucus in upper respiratory tract.	Digestive enzymes (lactase, isomaltase, lipase, etc.)
Asthma	Discontinued two-thirds asthma medications (per doctor) in one year due to elimination of inflammatory gluten and inhalant allergens.	Quercetin, natural anti-inflammatory agent to eliminate gut inflammation and improve airborne allergies
Multiple food allergies	Lowered "toxic burden" on immune system by elimination diet.	Zinc as an immune modulator Quercetin as natural anti-inflammatory/ antihistamine Custom vitamins

(continued on next page)

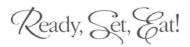

Daniel was diagnosed with gluten sensitivity per Faye's recommendation when he was five years old. Prior to his diagnosis he had always been in the fifth percentile on height and weight and was slow to gain weight. He weighed 32 pounds in kindergarten!

He also developed asthma, food allergies, and eczema and vomited often with no apparent cause. His entire family went on gluten-free diet after Daniel and his father were both diagnosed with gluten sensitivity. Within the first year, Daniel grew about five inches taller and gained ten pounds! Daniel's parents ran some food allergy testing (IgG, or delayed onset) which indicated multiple severe allergies. Since gluten sensitivity is an autoimmune disease, it overwhelms the person's immune system, which can lead to intestinal inflammation. As a result a single bite of an irritant such as egg or a dairy product could trigger allergic reactions, such as projectile vomiting in Daniel's case. This gut inflammation, per his allergy doctor, exacerbated his airway allergies. As Daniel's intestinal inflammation was improved by digestive enzymes and a gluten-free, dairy-free diet, his asthma improved markedly.

Five years later, Daniel weighs eighty-six pounds. He is a bright, happy, and healthy boy, enjoying school and playing linebacker on his football team.

Nutrition Foundation Program (NFP) for Autism Spectrum Disorders

Understanding Autism

Autism spectrum disorders (ASD) and pervasive developmental disorder (PDD) are broadly defined by many scientists as multifactorial dysfunction of neurotoxic, neuroimmune, neurometabolic systems. Autism spectrum disorders include multiple disorders from severe autism on the low end to Asperger's disorder on the high end of the spectrum.

According to Dr. Richard S. Lord, PhD, "The pathophysiology of ASD is likely to progress from increased oxidative challenge, . . . decreased glutathione status, immune dysregulation . . . and decreased methylation . . . . The net result is loss of neuronal integration necessary for normal perception and language ability and the onset of social withdrawal or self-stimulation behaviors." Here are some important facts to remember:

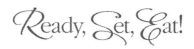

- The onset of autism spectrum disorders occurs during the first three years of life.
- More than two million Americans are currently affected by autism.
- According to the Center for Disease Control, between 1 in 80 and 1 in 240 children have ASDs, or an average of 1 in 110 eight-year-old children in the United States have an ASD.
- The U.S. population of autistic people ages 3 to 22 is 330,197. The estimated United States economic cost of caring for autistic children is $90,959,911,541. (source: **www.fightingautism.org**)
- Autistic children tend to suffer from co-morbid conditions such as sensory processing disorders, food allergies and intolerances, and heavy metal toxicity, further complicating their difficulties with learning, communicating, and relating—each exacerbating the other. Therefore, in order for children within the autism spectrum to emerge from this disorder, a combination of individualized occupational therapies, speech therapies, physical therapies, and nutritional therapies are necessary components of treatment. The following is a simplified illustration of the interconnections between autism, celiac disease, ADD, ADHD, sensory processing disorder, and food allergies and intolerances.

How do I test my child for ASD/PDD?

1. Seek the services of a developmental pediatrician immediately. If there is no developmental pediatrician, then work with a pediatrician with training in autism spectrum disorders (i.e., preferably Defeat Autism Now! [DAN] certified doctors) to diagnose ASD or PDD.
2. If the child is diagnosed with ASD/PDD, seek the services of a pediatric gastrointestinal doctor who is familiar with ASD/PDD, or a Defeat Autism Now! (DAN) doctor trained to perform biomedical testing. The autistic individual should be GI tested for proper digestion absorption, intestinal permeability, gut inflammation, gut dysbiosis (microbiota), and serum or urine toxic metal test.
3. Seek out the services of a nutritionist who specializes in autism and is knowledgeable in restoring gastrointestinal health as well as dietary and nutrition deficits.

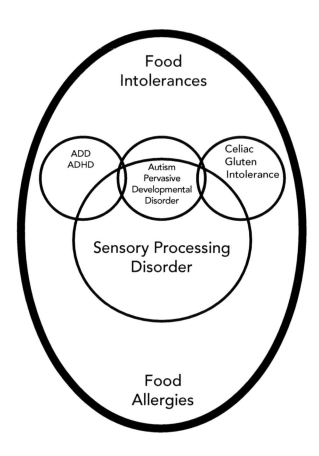

Food
Intolerances

ADD
ADHD

Autism
Pervasive
Developmental
Disorder

Celiac
Gluten
Intolerance

Sensory Processing
Disorder

Food
Allergies

What Parents of Children of ASD/PDD Need to Know

1. According to a new study published October 5, 2009, in the American
   Academy of Pediatrics' journal *Pediatrics*, a parent-reported autism
   prevalence rate is **1 in every 91 American children**, including **1 in
   58 boys**. The study used data gathered as part of the 2007 National Survey
   of Children's Health (NSCH), a national survey directed and funded by the
   Health Resources and Services Administration (HRSA) and Centers for
   Disease Control and Prevention (CDC).

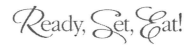

2. Autism spectrum disorders are treatable!
   • Identify the environmental triggers like mercury, aluminum, lead, and other toxic metal exposures like parent's work environment (radiation, chemicals).
   • There might be a genetic component in autism (gain of chromosome; inherited enzyme deficiencies).
   • Investigate traumatic events at the onset of autism such as premature birth, emergency C-sections, breach child, mother's infection, yeast overgrowth transferred by mother during childbirth, or viral infections.
   • Sulfation: Almost all people with autism have very high levels of sulfate in the urine which could cause a low glutathione status (glutathione is a critical antioxidant that clears the liver from toxins). This can be naturally reversed in time with customized multivitamins and minerals with free-form amino acids.
   • Methylation: Most children within the ASD are undermethylated due to insufficiency of sulfur donor amino acids such as GABA, or taurine, or glutathione. This is the reason why these children are not able to detoxify properly, thus creating a high body toxic burden. This can improve with custom multivitamins and minerals and proper ratios of amino acids.
   • In autism, TNF (tumor necrosis factor) is elevated, which can inhibit the conversion of cystein to sulfate.
   • Autism, according to many leading autism researchers, is a condition associated with multiple gastrointestinal issues. As an autism medical expert, Dr. Woody McGinnis would say, "Look below the diaphragm," referring to candida or viral damage causing a compromised intestinal lining. This in turn can lead to a leaky gut which can cause multiple food allergies and food intolerances (gluten, casein, oxalates, salicylates, phenols, amines). The sooner dietary intervention occurs, the faster the child's digestive tract is restored, and the sooner he/she will be able to emerge from autism. Yes—autism is treatable. The chart on page 38 indicates the prevalence of gastrointestinal issues in autism.

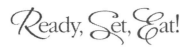

	Dr. McGinnis	Helena et al.
GI Issues		91% (siblings 25%, controls 0%)
Enterocolitis	88% (Ashwood)	
Esophagitis	69%	
Abdominal Pain	69%	46.6%
Duodenitis	67%	
Chronic Diarrhea	58%	75.6%
Gastritis	42%	
Constipation	35%	44.8%
Gas		55.2%
Abnormal Bowel		43%

McGinnis, "Defeat Autism Now," *McCartney Journal of Medical Microbiology* 2005; Ashwood, Journal of Clinical Immunology 2004 Nov;24(6): 664-73.

Mercury Toxicity and Autism

According to the EPA, the concern level of total mercury exposure per child from all sources is 0.1mcg/kg (microgram per kilogram) per day. For children who received vaccinations manufactured prior to 1999, on average 182.5 mcg of mercury from thimerosal alone was given in the first 6 months of a child's life. This exceeded the EPA levels of 126 mcg of mercury from *all sources* by 69 percent for a 6-month old baby.

How to Protect Yourself and Your Children from Toxic Metal Exposure

Although after 1999, per American Academy of Pediatrics' recommendations, pharmaceutical companies removed thimerosal from U.S. children's vaccines, other vaccines may still contain mercury, aluminum, and lead. Aluminum phosphate and aluminum hydroxide are widely used adjuvants (a substance used to enhance the body's response to antigens). In the first six months, vaccines, according to toxicology studies, can enter the brain and cause neurodegenerative disorders.

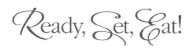

Read more about the potentially harmful vaccination preservatives at **www.vacinfo.org**. In the meantime, you can protect your child from exposure to toxic metal preservatives in vaccines by the following:

1) Reading vaccine ingredients, and specifically asking for a thimerosal-free alternative for these vaccines. For more information, visit: www.cdc.gov.

2) Sharing your concern on negative neurological side effects of **multiple** vaccines for your child with the pediatrician, as they will often offer an alternative vaccination schedule. To read more on sources of heavy metal toxicity in the environment visit: **www.specialneedsnutrition.com**.

The following table, as reported by Janet Raloff in her report, "Studies aim to resolve confusion over mercury risks from fish," indicates safe and unsafe sources of fish.

Guide to mercury levels in different varieties of fish and shellfish

LOW-MERCURY

VERY LOW	VERY LOW
Shrimp	Pollock
Sardines	Atlantic Mackerel
Tilapia	Anchovies, Sole, and Plaice
Oysters and Mussels	Crabs
Clams	Pike
Scallops	Butterfish
Salmon	Catfish
Crayfish	Squid
Freshwater Trout	Atlantic Croaker
Ocean Perch and Mullet	Whitefish

MODERATE-MERCURY

ABOVE AVERAGE	MODERATELY HIGH
Pacific Mackerel (Chub)	Carp and Buffalo Fish
Smelt	Halibut
Atlantic Tilefish	Sea Trout
Cod	Sablefish
Canned Light Tuna	Lingcod and Scorpionfish
Spiny Lobster	Sea Bass
Snapper, Porgy, Sheepshead	Pacific Croaker
Skate	American Lobster
Freshwater Perch	Freshwater Bass
Haddock, Hake, Monkfish	Bluefish

HIGH-MERCURY

HIGH	VERY HIGH
Canned Albacore Tuna	King Mackerel
Spanish Mackerel	Swordfish
Fresh/Frozen Tuna	Shark
Grouper	Gulf Tilefish
Marlin	Tuna Sushi/Bluefin Tuna
Orange Roughy	

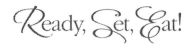

Nutrition Foundation Program (NFP) for ASD

Please review the 6 steps of NFP described on page 14, and the additional steps on page 29, which are useful in managing ASD.

> 1. **Limit the daily sugar intake to 30 grams (6 teaspoons) for children and 40 grams (8 teaspoons) for adults.**
> 2. **Reduce fast food intake from daily to occasionally.**
> 3. **Eliminate food allergens and excitotoxins (phenols in artificial colors and flavors).**
> 4. **Add high-quality multivitamin/mineral supplements (best if customized).**
> 5. **Add a high-quality probiotic.**
> 6. **Add a high-quality fish oil.**
> 7. **Eliminate gluten (grain protein).**
> 8. **Eliminate casein (dairy protein).**
> 9. **Add digestive enzymes.**
> 10. **Add amino acids as needed.**

Case Studies

Ben: 4.5-year-old boy

Diagnosed with encephalopathy manifested by pervasive developmental disorder and autism spectrum disorder

Before Ben's birth, his mother was prescribed strong drugs for extreme nausea (hyperemesis gravidarum) and for low back pain, as well as an inducing drug. Starting the second night of birth: Ben would scream and cry for hours on end! After a few months, Ben was diagnosed with colic and gastro-esophageal reflux disease (GERD), and a strong antacid was prescribed, then a stronger one until 15 months. Ben was not a happy toddler, did not make good eye contact, and although he did meet *most* of his typical milestones, he was always agitated. By age two, Ben was having facial rashes and eczema. The same year, he received his MMR (measles, mumps, rubella) vaccines along with two flu shots which coincided with more tantrums. Ben was nonverbal, stopped responding to his name, and became isolated, sometimes banging his head on the furniture. Ben

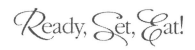

was unfortunately a case of a baby born with a high toxic burden, which probably triggered his colic and later GERD for which more drugs were prescribed, adding insult to injury. With careful monitoring of his stool, we could find the right pre- and probiotic to aid in restoring the gut flora he so desperately needed to rebuild his immunity and to synthesize B vitamins that eventually helped reduce his tantrums. Mom was also careful about not offering salicylates (red grapes, apples, berries, citrus, cucumbers, and peppers), and oxalates (almonds, soy, beans, spinach, and beets). By age 3.5, after implementing the NFP with other therapies, Ben made consistent progress in all 5 areas of expressive speech (100-plus words in 6 months), eye contact, normal sleep, and socialization.

Before NFP and custom vitamin/mineral supplements	After NFP and custom vitamin/mineral supplements (gluten & dairy free)	Nutritional Supplementation Program
Head banging	Improved by 80% with gluten, casein, and soy elimination and low-oxalate diet.	Improved 100% Magnesium to relax the nervous system
Asocial behaviors Physical aggression Tantrums	Elimination of preservatives, coloring, and additives. Lower sugar, yeast free diet, low oxalates, low salicylates (aspirin-like substances).	Taurine, nondairy single strain probiotics
Delayed expressive speech	Improved by 50% with gluten and dairy elimination which caused inflammation as well as concentration, sensory and modulation deficits.	Dimethyl glycine, Carnitine, B6 along with other B1-2-3-5-12-Folate, vitamins
Chronic diarrhea	Improved by 75%–80% after yeast-free diet followed & allergens and intolerances eliminated.	1 Trillion + probiotics, digestive enzymes, prebiotics, limited protein

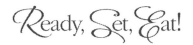

Ray: 3.5-year-old boy

Diagnosed with pervasive developmental disorder

Before custom vitamin/ mineral supplements and NFP	After custom vitamin/ mineral supplements and NFP (gluten & dairy free)	Nutritional Supplementation Program
Lack of eye contact	Improved by 80% after gluten, casein, and soy elimination.	Improved 100% with fatty acid supplement (DHA Jr.)
Daily tantrums	Preservatives, coloring, additives, yeast-free, lower sugar diet	Nondairy multiple strain probiotics
Delayed expressive language	Speaks 250-plus words after start of gluten and dairy elimination.	Dimethyl glycine Carnitine, B6 along with B1-2-3-5-12-Folate Fatty acid supplement
Chronic Constipation	Improved by 90% after elimination of food allergens and intolerances.	100-plus billion dairy-free probiotics, digestive enzymes, prebiotics, limited proteins, custom minerals
Anxiety, agitation	Improved by 25% with elimination of gluten, casein, soy, and salicylates.	Taurine, methionine, selenium, L-Tyrosine

At the two-year well visit to the pediatrician, Ray spoke only ten words, had chronic constipation, occasionally flapped his hands in excitement and frequently had tantrums.

At 2.5 years, a speech therapist noticed speech delays, white tongue, dry patches on the skin, profuse sweating, and casein and gluten food intolerances. At 2.6 years, a month after starting a gluten-free, casein-free, and yeast-free diet,

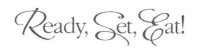

Ray started to engage in play activities for longer periods, listened well, and even verbally requested that his Mom play his favorite CD.

At 2.7 years, Ray danced and laughed out loud for the first time at the circus!

About six months after the start of NFP, he consistently progressed in all five areas: perfect eye contact; great socialization with one very short tantrum every three to four weeks; finishes longer tasks in therapy sessions; does not run away; and speaks over 250 words.

Nutrition Foundation Program (NFP) for Attention Deficit Disorder (ADD) and Hyperactivity Disorder (ADHD)

Understanding ADD and ADHD

Unlike hypoglycemia, where a blood test can prove the diagnosis, there is no lab test that can objectively diagnose ADD or ADHD. To further complicate matters, the main symptoms of ADD and ADHD such as inattention, fidgety behavior, hyperactivity, impulsivity, and inability to finish tasks are present in most children from time to time. To define a child's behavior as a sign of ADD or ADHD, pediatricians and mental health professionals must rely on parents' and teachers' observations of the child's behaviors in comparison to other children their age.

In recent years, the scientific community has developed alternative biomedical interventions for treating ADD and ADHD that are promising. Of course, psychotherapy is always useful in coping with the symptoms associated with ADD and ADHD. The following facts give a perspective to the ever-growing epidemic of ADHD in the U.S.:

- Much like autism, ADHD involves dysfunctions of the immune system, the nervous system, and the digestive system.
- Up to 10 percent of the children in U.S. are believed to have symptoms of ADHD.
- About 25 percent of children with ADHD suffer from sleep apnea.
- About 3 million children in the U.S. are currently taking ADHD medications.
- About 1.5 million adults in the U.S. are currently taking ADHD medications; this number has doubled since 2000.

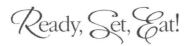

- The cost of treating ADHD is approximately $3 billion.
- The growth of autism seems to be correlated with the growth of ADHD.
- There are dietary and nutritional interventions for ADHD that are able to produce 80 to 90 percent positive outcomes (see ADHD case studies).

Nine Signs and Symptoms of ADHD

1. Not giving close attention
2. Difficulty sustaining attention
3. Not listening when spoken to
4. Not following instructions
5. Difficulty organizing tasks
6. Avoiding engaging in mentally hard tasks
7. Easily distracted
8. Forgetful in daily activities
9. Losing things

What Parents of ADD and ADHD children should know

1. ADD and ADHD individuals commonly suffer from the following vitamin deficiencies: vitamin A; thiamin or B1; and folate, the deficiency of which is associated with nervousness, and hyperactivity. The person's deficiencies should be restored through natural vitamin therapy as vitamin deficiency symptoms can mimic ADD and ADHD symptoms.

2. ADD and ADHD individuals also can have neurotransmitter insufficiencies which are chemicals that relay nerve messages. There are two main types of neurotransmitters: excitatory and inhibitory. Maintaining the balance between the excitatory and inhibitory neurotransmitters is key to an optimal neurotransmitter program. Since there is a curtain of blood called the blood-brain barrier that wraps around the brain, the neurotransmitters taken orally cannot cross this barrier. However, customizing the right vitamins and minerals along with free-form amino acids (protein) is the basis of our NFP program which has offered a natural alternative to a drug based ADD/ADHD program.

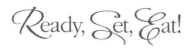

3. Explore the body's toxic burden from either the external environment (air pollution) or internal environment (mercury in vaccines, pesticides on food).

4. Investigate previous antibiotic usage to discover collateral gastrointestinal symptoms.

5. Test presence of yeast or fungi as a source of leaky gut which could be causing severe food allergies or intolerances with physical and psychological side effects.

Nutrition Foundation Program (NFP) for ADD and ADHD:

To read the details of my NFP protocol refer to page 14, and pages 29,30 and 31 that are applicable to ADD, ADHD.

1. *Limit the daily sugar intake to 30 grams (6 teaspoons) for children and 40 grams (8 teaspoons) for adults.*
2. *Reduce fast food intake from daily to occasionally.*
3. *Eliminate food allergens and excitotoxins (phenols in artificial colors and flavors).*
4. *Add customized high-quality multivitamin/mineral supplements.*
5. *Add a high-quality probiotic.*
6. *Add a high-quality fish oil.*
7. *Eliminate gluten (grain protein).*
8. *Eliminate casein (dairy protein).*
9. *Add digestive enzymes.*
10. *Add amino acids as needed.*

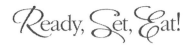

Case Studies

Carter: 17-year-old young man

Diagnosed with attention deficit disorder (ADD) in 1999
and gluten sensitivity in 2009

Before custom vitamin/ mineral supplements and NFP	After custom vitamin/ mineral supplements and NFP (gluten & dairy free)	Customized Nutritional Supplementation Program
Severe anxiety, difficulty transitioning between activities	Improved by 50% shortly following elimination of gluten.	Improved 75% with high magnesium sulfate to relax the nervous system
Lack of concentration	Elimination of preservatives, coloring, additives and lower sugar	Zinc citrate to help with concentration Nondairy probiotic
Constipation	Improved by 50% with gluten elimination.	Digestive enzymes (lactase, isomaltase, lipase, etc.)
Multiple food allergies	Lowered toxic burden on immune system by elimination of gluten, dairy, MSG, and artificial coloring.	Zinc citrate as an immune modulator
Inability to focus on complex tasks (such as math problems)	Able to improve grades from B's to A's in math without two ADD medications while on gluten-free diet.	Multivitamins with high B vitamins, zinc, and magnesium to aid memory and retention and alleviate severe anxiety
Anxiety, inattention	Improved by 75% after gluten-free diet.	5-HTP Hydroxy tryptophan

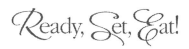

Carter came to us at 16, slightly overweight, with neck twitching thought to be Tourett's syndrome, inattention, and severe acne he had since the age of 6! He took four ADD drugs which his loving mother and Carter both agreed were helpful only part of the day.

He started with dietary changes like eliminating gluten, casein, and three other food allergens. Results were astonishing: more attentiveness, less anxiety, and more regular bowels. Next he took customized multivitamin/mineral supplements and free-form amino acids to help bridge the nutritional gap shown by biomedical tests. This led to improved math grades and 80 percent reduction of acne signs, as well as elimination of neck twitching! Six months into the Nutrition Foundation Program, Carter's focus improved, and he no longer needed his four ADD meds. He successfully finished 11th grade with all A's and his acne was eliminated. A year later, he was drug-free, with 100 points higher on his SAT writing score.

Meghan: 9-year-old girl
Diagnosed with attention deficit hyperactivity disorder (ADHD)

Meghan was a normal third grader who has just turned nine when she came to our clinic. She was naturally outgoing: however, she has difficulty focusing and staying calm, and was thus diagnosed with ADHD at age six for which she was prescribed two prescription medications.

Meghan's breath was at times sour, leading her parents to seek help. Shortly after the initial assessment, Meghan was put on a low-sugar, gluten-free diet in addition to strong probiotics to help restore her gut health while waiting the results of the organic acid urine test. The first week on the diet, her parents reported calmer behavior and fewer stomach aches. She has become proficient at reading food labels at the store. Gradually, after three months on the custom vitamin/mineral supplements, Meghan's parents decided to wean her from her ADHD drugs. After six months on the NFP, Meghan is medication-free, a testimony to using proper nutrition and familial and emotional support in restoring a child's health.

(continued on next page)

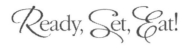

Meghan: 9-year-old girl

Before custom vitamin/ mineral supplements and NFP	After custom vitamin/ mineral supplements and NFP (gluten & dairy free)	Customized Nutritional Supplementation Program
Severe anxiety, difficulty transitioning between activities	Improved by 50% shortly after elimination of gluten.	Improved 75%. High magnesium sulfate to relax the nervous system.
Lack of concentration	Elimination of preservatives, coloring, additives, and lower sugar.	Zinc citrate to help with concentration Nondairy probiotic
Constipation	Improved by 50% with gluten elimination.	Digestive enzymes (lactase, isomaltase, lipase, etc.)
Multiple food allergies	Lowered toxic burden on immune system by elimination of gluten, dairy, MSG, and artificial coloring.	Zinc citrate as an immune modulator
Inability to focus on complex tasks (such as math problems)	Able to improve grades from B's to A's in math without two ADD medications while on gluten-free diet.	Multivitamins with high B vitamins, zinc, and magnesium to aid memory and retention and alleviate severe anxiety

Part II: Recipe Guide

Valentine's Day Menu

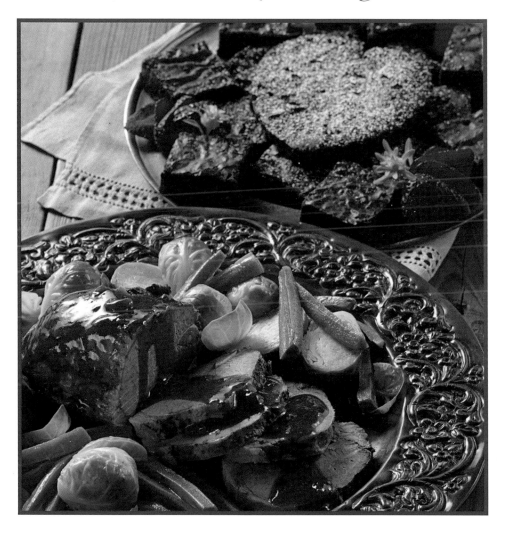

Beef Roast with Brussels Sprouts and Baby Carrots,
Easy and Elegant Brownies

Thanksgiving Holiday Menu

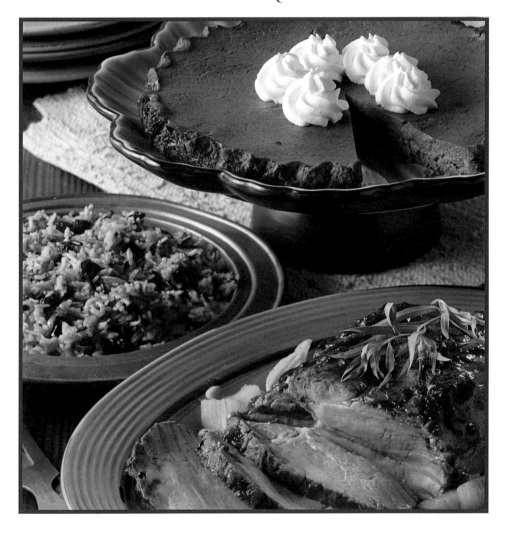

*Roasted Pork Tenderloin with Mango-Ginger Chutney,
Almond and Cranberry Rice, Pumpkin Chiffon Pie*

Christmas Holiday Menu

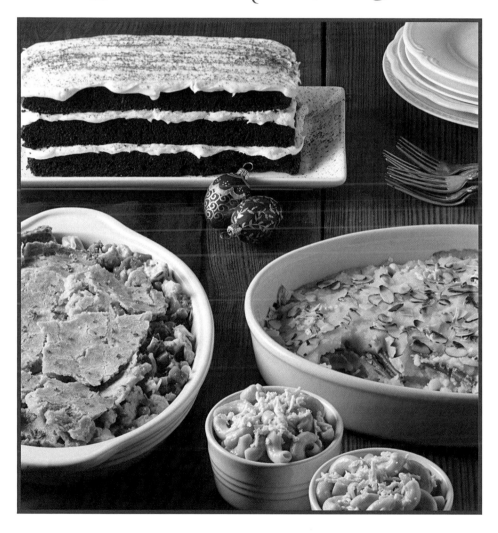

Chicken Pot Pie, Bûche de Noël, Faye's Green Bean Casserole,
Organic Rice Macaroni and Cheese

Breakfast & Snacks

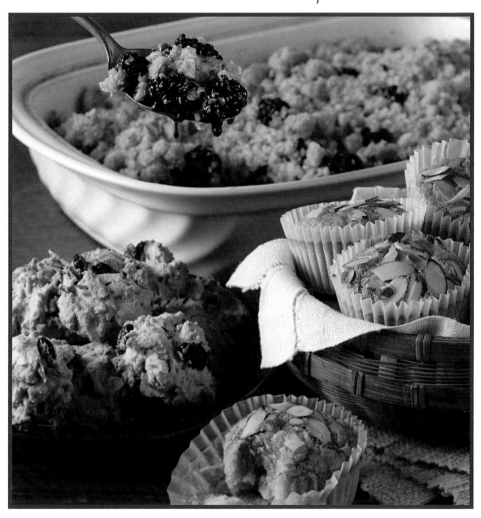

Scrumptious Cranberry Cookies, Berry Crumble, Perfect Vanilla Cupcakes

Midday Meal

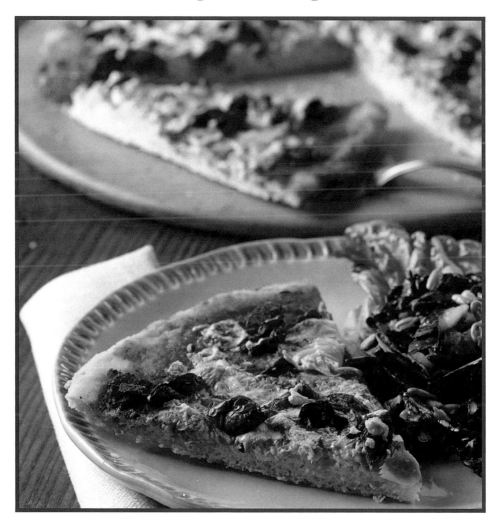

Miniature Sausage Pizzas, Red Cabbage and Onion Salad

Dinner Delight

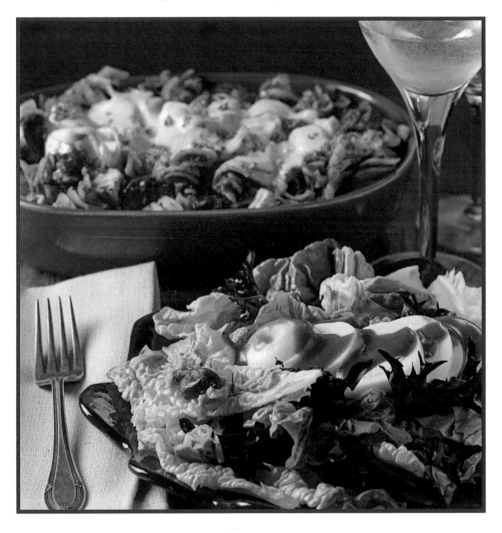

Exotic Salad Niçoise, Baked Ziti

Desserts

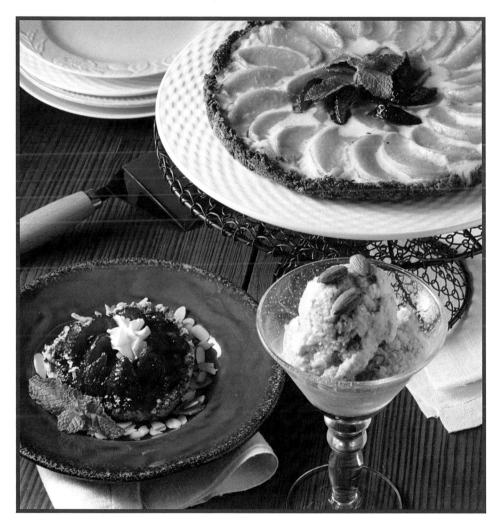

Fresh Strawberry Pie, Custard Peach Pie, Silky Coconut Ice Cream

The Sensory Diet

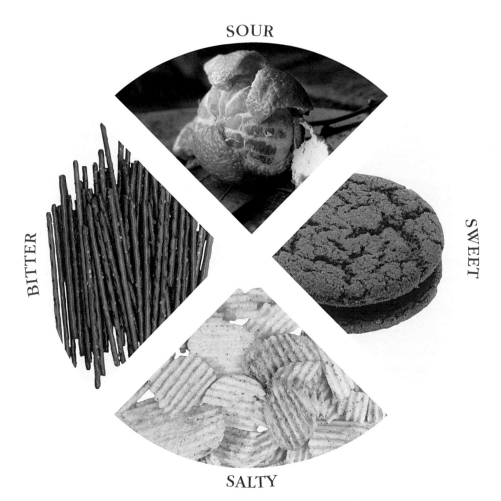

SOUR

SWEET

SALTY

BITTER

Example of the tastes that stimulate the underdeveloped mouth.

Plan on stimulating the mouth with four tastes daily:
Salty (Lay's Stax Potato Chips); sour (tangerine, drops of lime juice); sweet
(cookies); bitter (gluten-free pretzels). See page 24 for more details.

Menu Plans and Recipes

Breakfast, Breads, and Snacks
66–79

Soups, Salads, and Sides
80–95

Beef, Pork, Poultry, Seafood, and Meatless Mains
96–115

Cookies and Desserts
116–133

An asterisk (*) in the ingredient list denotes a product you can find on the Shopping Guide on page 134.

Recipe designators, such as gluten-free, casein-free, yeast-free, etc., are listed below the recipes.

All ingredients vary according to product availability. This book does not make any guarantees as to the safety of ingredients in commercial foods for people with food allergies or sensitivities and intolerances.

The information contained in this book is not intended to diagnose or cure any disease.

WEEK 1

	Sunday	Monday	Tuesday
Breakfast	Mouthwatering Crepes with Fresh Berries and coconut yogurt* 1 cup unsweetened vanilla almond milk*	Lip-Smacking French Toast with Cinnamon Hormone-free bacon 1 cup cultured coconut milk*	Apple cinnamon cereal* 1 cup hemp milk*
Snack	1/2 cup Mineral-Packed Trail Mix Water	1 medium pear Water	1 Crunchy Granola Bar Water
Lunch	Creamy Cauliflower and Broccoli Soup 10–12 Seattle crackers* or plain rice crackers	Brown rice tortilla* with GF deli meat*, lettuce, olives, and avocado slices Celery sticks with fruit dip	Hearty Vegetarian Tacos Mixed Dark Green Salad with Avocado Dressing
Lunchbox	Weekend, not needed	Same as above	Crispy Chicken Nuggets Celery sticks filled with organic cashew or almond butter 1 cup applesauce
Snack	1 apple with small portion of fruit dip	1/2 cup Mineral-Packed Trail Mix Water	Blue corn chips* Hummus dip
Dinner	Vegetable Lasagna Endive Salad with Parisian Vinaigrette Seattle crackers*	Crispy Salmon Nuggets Baked potato Baked Spaghetti Squash	Manicotti Red Cabbage and Onion Salad
Dessert	1 cup Fruit Salad with Crunchy Topping	1 cup Tapioca Coconut Pudding	1 scoop Silky Coconut Ice Cream

*See Shopping Guide on page 134. Legend key: GF (gluten-free)

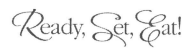

Wednesday	Thursday	Friday	Saturday
GF Rice Chex Cereal* 1 cup cultured coconut milk*	Coconut Lava 1 cup unsweetened vanilla almond milk*	Wake-Up-Your-Brain Shake Green tea (decaffeinated)	Herbed Scrambled Eggs Hormone-free bacon 1 cup unsweetened vanilla almond milk*
1 cup Piña Colada Shake Water	10-12 rice chips* Hummus dip Water	1 medium fruit Water	1 almond coconut bar* Water
Exotic Salad Niçoise 6–8 Seattle crackers*	Crispy Salmon Nuggets Jungle Salad	Brown rice tortilla* with GF deli meat*, lettuce, olives, and avocado Cut-up fresh bell pepper (red, yellow, or green) with fruit dip	Veggie Burger Burritos 1 serving organic navy beans 10–12 rice chips*
Same as above Fresh sour apple pieces with fruit dip	Crispy Salmon Nuggets Rice chips* Ranch dressing/dip 4–5 baby carrots	Same as above	Weekend, not needed
10–12 rice chips* 1 tablespoon almond or cashew butter*	1 hemp sunflower seed bar* Water	10–15 rice chips* Hummus dip	Avocado Dip 10–12 rice chips*
Chicken Pot Pie Jungle Salad with Avocado Dressing	Beef Roast with Brussels Sprouts and Baby Carrots Chilled Cucumber and Red Onion Salad	Crispy Chicken Nuggets Roasted Vegetables Creamy Snappy Guacamole with rice chips	Cod with Spinach and Tomatoes Quinoa Linguini Alfredo
1 cup cultured coconut yogurt with chopped pecans	1 scoop Delightful Ice Cream	1 cup coconut yogurt with crunchy pecan topping	1 slice Fresh Strawberry Pie

WEEK 2

	Sunday	Monday	Tuesday
Breakfast	Bacon-Tomato Mini Crustless Quiches Sweet Potato Hash Browns 1 cup hemp milk	1 cup organic maple buckwheat flakes * 1 cup unsweetened vanilla almond milk	1 cup Piña Colada Shake 1 cup hemp milk or raw unhomogenized milk
Snack	1/2 cup Mineral-Packed Trail Mix Water	1 Rice Crispy Ball* Water	1 medium pear or peach Water
Lunch	Rolled up GF turkey slices 1 plate organic vegetables with vinaigrette (celery, baby carrots, cucumber, zucchini)	Pork Tenderloin slices (leftover from Sunday) wrapped in a brown rice tortilla	Crispy Chicken Nuggets* House salad with vinaigrette
Lunchbox	Weekend, not needed	Same as above	Sliced Hot Dogs* Zucchini, bell pepper strips, celery, and baby carrots with ranch dip
Snack	1 Perfect Vanilla Cupcake 1 cup unsweetened almond milk	1 almond and coconut bar*	1 medium fruit (low-glycemic, pear, grapefruit)
Dinner	Roasted Pork Tenderloin with Mango-Chutney Roasted Asparagus and Cinammon Sweet Potatoes	Antibiotic-free hot dogs* GF hot dog buns* Chilled Cucumber and Red Onion Salad	Savory Butternut Squash Soup Flaky Buttermilk Biscuits
Dessert	1 roasted pear	8 animal cookies*	Rice Pudding with granola topping*

*See Shopping Guide on page 134. Legend key: GF (gluten-free)

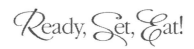

Wednesday	Thursday	Friday	Saturday
Coconut Oatmeal* 1 cup unsweetened vanilla almond milk	1 cup creamy rice cereal* made with 1 cup unsweetened vanilla almond milk served with GF granola topping* 1 cup almond milk	2 GF waffles* 1 teaspoon organic blue agave nectar* or raw unfiltered local honey (gfcfef) 1 cup hemp milk	Lip-Smacking French Toast with Cinnamon Canadian Bacon* 1 cup Berry Shake
10–12 rice crackers* Hummus dip Water	8–10 baby carrots Avocado Dip Water	1 hemp-sunflower seed bar Water	1 sliced apple with cashew or almond butter* Water
Crispy Salmon Nuggets 5–6 sweet potato fries 1 bowl Jungle Salad with Lemon Vinaigrette 8 animal cookies*	Brown rice tortilla* with bacon, organic lettuce , avocado, and olives Celery sticks with ranch dip	Hearty Vegetarian Tacos Jungle Salad 1 cup Creamy Snappy Guacamole 8 animal cookies*	Italian Meatballs with brown rice spaghetti* Quick and Tasty Garlic Toast
Turkey slices with rice chips* and baby carrots 1 small cultured coconut yogurt	Same as above	Brown rice tortilla* with GF deli meat* 1/4 cup roasted lightly salted edamame	Weekend, not needed
1 cup papaya	1 cup organic berries with cultured coconut yogurt*	10–12 rice chips* Hummus dip	1 cup GF cereal with 1 cup hemp milk or unsweetened almond milk or water
Exotic Salad Niçoise 1 bowl cauliflower soup	Oven-Roasted Halibut Roasted Vegetables	Scrumptious Beef Kabobs Saffron Rice	Creamy Sweet Potato Soup 10–12 Seattle crackers* 1 cup dinner salad with Avocado Dressing
1 cup Tapioca Coconut Pudding	1 cup cultured coconut yogurt*	1 cup Fruit Salad with Crunchy Topping	1 scoop Silky Coconut Ice Cream with organic strawberries

WEEK 3

	Sunday	Monday	Tuesday
Breakfast	Florentine Omelet with tomato and chives 1/2 cup fresh-squeezed juice	1 cup high-protein shake 100% egg white protein powder 1 cup unsweetened vanilla almond milk*	GF savory sausage* Herbed Scrambled Eggs 1/2 cup fresh-squeezed juice
Snack	1 organic fruit	1/2 cup Mineral-Packed Trail Mix	1 cup Fruit Salad with Crunchy Topping
Lunch	Juicy Hamburger with pickle and tomato 10–12 GF waffle fries*	Hot dogs with GF hot dog buns Red, yellow, or green bell pepper chunks 4–5 rice chips	Bacon-Tomato Mini Crustless Quiches Cut-up English cucumbers with organic sea salt
Lunchbox	Weekend, not needed	Same as above	Same as above
Snack	10–12 raw soaked walnuts or almonds*	1 organic fruit	1 cup coconut yogurt
Dinner	1 bowl Energy-Packed Bone Stock 10–12 Seattle crackers*	Miniature Sausage Pizzas Mixed Dark Green Salad	Chicken Pot Pie 1 cup cole slaw with vinaigrette
Dessert	1 slice Custard Peach Pie	8 animal cookies*	1 Easy and Elegant Brownie

*See Shopping Guide on page 134. Legend key: GF (gluten-free)

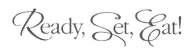

Wednesday	Thursday	Friday	Saturday
2 buckwheat waffles 2 slices Canadian bacon 1 cup cultured coconut milk*	Mineral-Rich Shake 1–2 slices GF toast with cashew butter Water	Mango Orange Shake 1–2 slices GF toast* with sunflower butter*	1 cup Berry Rich Breakfast Risotto 1/4 cup GF granola topping 4–5 walnut halves 1 cup hemp milk*
Pretzels* with fruit dip	1 organic fruit	1 hemp sunflower bar*	10–12 raw soaked walnuts or almonds*
Juicy Hamburger with cheese (made on Sunday, from the freezer) Endive Salad with Parisian Vinaigrette	Miniature Sausage Pizzas Organic celery & carrot sticks	Chicken Potato Salad 10–12 rice chips*	Vegetarian Tacos
2 slices bread* with GF deli meat*, lettuce, and tomato 10–12 rice chips	Same as above	Same as above	Weekend, not needed
Hummus dip with rice chips	1 cup Fruit Salad with Crunchy Topping	Celery sticks with ranch dip	Sliced English cucumber with organic sea salt
Oven-Roasted Mackerel Millet and Asapargus	Lemon Olive Chicken Roasted Vegetables	Crispy Salmon Nuggets Endive Salad with Lemon Vinaigrette Baked Sweet Potatoes in Syrup	Italian Meatballs Mixed Dark Green Salad with Avocado Dressing
1 hemp sunflower bar*	1 cup Fruit Salad with Crunchy Topping	1/2 cup Rice Pudding with granola topping*	1/2 cup Berry Sorbet with chopped organic pecans

WEEK 4

	Sunday	Monday	Tuesday
Breakfast	High-Energy Frittata 1 cup unsweetened vanilla almond milk*	Herbed Scrambled Eggs 2 slices whole grain bread* with 1/2 cup fresh-squeezed juice	Skinny Berry Shake 1 slice Lip-Smacking French Toast with Cinnamon
Snack	1 cup Fruit Salad with Crunchy Topping	1–2 rice cakes* with 1 tablespoon organic almond butter*	1 organic apple
Lunch	Saffron Chicken Kabobs Almond and Cranberry Rice Endive Salad with Avocado Dressing Ginger lemonade	Veggie Burger Burritos Organic carrots and celery with Avocado Dip 1 French Madeleine	Artichoke Soup in a Flash Quick and Tasty Garlic Toast
Lunchbox	Weekend, not needed	Same as above	2 slices whole grain bread* 3–4 slices GF deli meat* 2 cucumber strips
Snack	10–12 raw soaked almonds or walnuts	1/2 cup Mineral-Packed Trail Mix	1 banana with 1 tablespoon almond butter
Dinner	Vegetable Lasagna Mixed Dark Green Salad with Avocado Dressing	Lemon Olive Chicken Quick and Tasty Garlic Toast	Beef Roast with Brussels Sprouts and Baby Carrots
Dessert	1 cup raspberry sorbet	1 cup Tapioca Coconut Pudding	1/2 cup Rice Pudding

*See Shopping Guide on page 134. Legend key: GF (gluten-free)

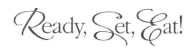

Wednesday	Thursday	Friday	Saturday
Coconut Lava 1/2 cup fresh-squeezed juice	1 GF waffles 1 tablespoon organic almond butterr* 1 cup hemp milk*	1 cup crunchy flax cereal* 1 cup Piña Colada Shake	Berry Rich Breakfast Risotto 1 cup unsweetened vanilla almond milk*
6 ounces cultured coconut yogurt*	1 organic fruit	1/2 cup Mineral-Packed Trail Mix	Ginger lemonade
2 medium corn tortilla wraps with deli chicken* and Avocado Dip	4–6 Crispy Chicken Nuggets Flaky Buttermilk Biscuits Organic green, yellow, and red bell pepper chunks with Avocado Dip	Brown rice tortillas with Scrumptious Beef Kabobs Chilled Cucumber and Red Onion Salad	Barbecue-Roasted Chicken Wings and Drumsticks GF waffle fries Red Cabbage and Onion Salad with Parisian Vinaigrette
Same as above	Same as above	Same as above (substitute Cucumber Salad with carrot and celery sticks with Avocado Dip)	Weekend, not needed
10–12 rice chips with hummus dip	10–12 pretzel* Cucumber dip	4–5 organic celery ribs 1 tablespoon organic almond butter or sun butter*	Creamy Snappy Guacamole with rice chips
Saffron Chicken Kabobs Red Cabbage and Onion Salad with Lemon Vinaigrette	Scrumptious Beef Kabobs Saffron Rice Mixed Dark Green Salad with Lemon Vinaigrette	Crispy Chicken Parmesan and Pasta Primavera with Vegetables Chilled Cucumber and Red Onion Salad	Roasted Turkey Baked Spaghetti Squash Cucumber dip
8 animal cookies*	1 cup cultured coconut yogurt* with chopped organic pecans	1 cup Fruit Salad with Crunchy Topping	Coconut Ice Cream Sandwich

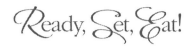

Breakfast, Breads, and Snacks

The Recipes

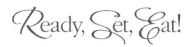

Mouthwatering Crêpes with Fresh Berries

Preparation Time: 5 minutes   *Cooking Time: 10 minutes*

1   tablespoon cooking oil
1/2 cup Gluten-Free Flour Blend (below)
1   pinch of organic sea salt
1/2 cup plain rice milk

1   free-range egg
1   cup fresh or frozen organic berries
Confectioners' sugar to taste

Heat the oil in a shallow nonstick skillet over medium heat. Mix the Flour Blend and next 4 ingredients in a bowl and whisk until smooth. Pour 1 ladle of the batter in the center of the skillet and immediately rotate the skillet until a thin layer of batter covers the bottom. Cook for 1 minute. Flip the crêpe with a wide flat spatula to prevent tearing. Cook for 1 minute or until golden on both sides. Repeat with remaining batter. Roll up the crêpes to enclose some of the berries in each and arrange on serving plates. Sprinkle with confectioners' sugar. *Serves 4*

Gluten-Free Flour Blend

1 3/4 cups white rice flour
1 1/4 cups brown rice flour

3/4 cup potato starch
1   cup tapioca starch

Combine the rice flours and starches in a large bowl and mix until well blended. Store in an airtight container. *Makes 4 3/4 cups*

| *Gluten-free* | *Casein-free* | *Yeast-free* | *Nut-free* |

Lip-Smacking French Toast with Cinnamon

Preparation Time: 15 minutes   *Cooking Time: 5 minutes*

1   free-range egg
1/3 cup plain rice milk
1   pinch of organic sea salt
4   thick slices gluten-free sandwich bread*

1   tablespoon cooking oil
1   tablespoon beet sugar
Cinnamon to taste

Beat the egg, rice milk and salt in a large flat-bottom bowl. Dip 1 slice of bread at a time in the milk mixture to coat both sides of the bread. Heat the oil in a large shallow skillet over medium heat. Place the bread slices 2 at a time in the skillet. Cook for 1 to 2 minutes on each side or until golden. Sprinkle with the beet sugar and cinnamon. *Serves 4*

Variation: Serve with creamy organic almond butter for an additional three grams of protein and eight grams of high-quality fatty acids per tablespoon.

| *Gluten-free* | *Casein-free* | *Yeast-free* | *Nut-free* |

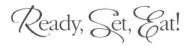

Herbed Scrambled Eggs

Preparation Time: 5 minutes   *Cooking Time: 5 minutes*

1 tablespoon extra-virgin olive oil	2 teaspoons gluten-free
4 free-range eggs, beaten	herbes de Provence*
1 tablespoon water	Organic sea salt to taste

Heat the oil in a nonstick skillet over medium heat for 1 minute. Whisk the eggs and remaining ingredients together. Pour the egg mixture into the heated skillet. Stir with a wooden spatula often until the mixture is soft but firm. **Serves 2**

Note: This is a basic low-carb, high-protein egg recipe that is easy and elegant. My children learned to cook very young by making this recipe on weekends.

Gluten-free	*Casein-free*	*Soy-free*	*Yeast-free*	*Nut-free*

High-Energy Frittata

Preparation Time: 10 minutes   *Cooking Time: 8 minutes*

4 cherry tomatoes	1/2 cup chopped yellow onion
2 strips gluten-free bacon, cooked	1/2 cup chopped zucchini
1 tablespoon extra-virgin olive oil	Organic sea salt and black pepper
3 large free-range eggs	to taste

Cut the cherry tomatoes into halves. Crumble the bacon strips into bite-size pieces. Heat the oil in a nonstick skillet over medium heat. Whisk the eggs and add the vegetables and bacon. Pour the egg mixture into the skillet. Cook for 4 minutes or until set around the edges. Cover and cook for 3 to 4 minutes or until the top is firm. Season with salt and pepper and serve. **Makes 2 small servings**

Note: This is a perfect breakfast to have about two hours before a work-out session because it offers sustained energy. For those who are on a low-fat diet, use one whole egg and three egg whites and two ounces of turkey bits instead of bacon.

Gluten-free	*Casein-free*	*Yeast-free*	*Nut-free*

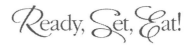

Florentine Omelet

Preparation Time: 10 minutes   Cooking Time: 20 minutes

1 strip gluten-free bacon
6 large free-range eggs
2 tablespoons organic coconut milk*
1/2 teaspoon organic sea salt
2 tablespoons butter substitute*
1/2 red bell pepper, finely chopped
1/2 yellow bell pepper, finely chopped
1/2 small yellow onion, finely chopped
1/2 cup (2 ounces) shredded Cheddar-flavor nondairy cheese*

Cook the bacon in a small skillet over medium heat. Drain on a paper towel; cool and crumble. Wipe the skillet. Beat the eggs, coconut milk and salt with a fork in a small bowl until well mixed. Melt half the butter in the skillet over medium-high heat until the butter turns color. Pour in the egg mixture. Cook until the edges turn golden and are set, about 10 seconds. Use a wooden spatula to stir the middle and pull the cooked edges toward the center. Cook 5 more seconds to help set the omelet, but do not overcook as it needs to be moist on top. Heat the remaining tablespoon butter in another small skillet over medium heat. Add the vegetables and cook until the onion is soft, stirring constantly. Add the bacon and cheese to the vegetable mixture. Spoon the vegetable filling over one side of the omelet. Slide the omelet onto a plate filled side first. Invert the pan swiftly to fold the other side over the filling. Serve warm. ***Serves 4***

Note: This is a high-protein, high-fat, low-carb breakfast that is nonfattening if eaten as a complement to other high-protein, low-animal fat, low-carb meals the rest of the day. Children or adults who are underweight or active could enjoy this meal at any time of the day to repair their cells while renewing their energy.

Gluten-free	*Casein-free*	*Soy-free*	*Yeast-free*	*Nut-free*

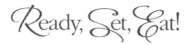
Bacon-Tomato Mini Crustless Quiches

Preparation Time: 15 minutes   *Cooking Time: 45 minutes*

1 slice gluten-free bacon*	3/4 cup chopped tomato
4 free-range eggs	1/2 cup nondairy sour cream*
2 tablespoons nondairy butter substitute*	1 cup grated nondairy cheese*
	1/4 teaspoon organic sea salt

Preheat the oven to 350 degrees. Cook the bacon in a skillet. Drain on a paper towel and chop into small bits. Beat the eggs in a medium bowl. Stir in the bacon and remaining ingredients. Pour into greased miniature muffin cups. Bake for 45 minutes or until a knife inserted in the center comes out clean. Serve warm. *Serves 6 to 8*

Note: These mini quiches are the whole family's favorite snack or breakfast. If allergic to soy, omit the sour cream. This fits perfectly in a moderate-fat, moderate-protein, low-carb, disaccharide-free meal plan.

Gluten-free	*Casein-free*	*Yeast-free*

Coconut Oatmeal

Preparation Time: 10 minutes   *Cooking Time: 10 minutes*

2 cups water	2 cups or 4 packets gluten-free
1/3 cup organic coconut milk*	instant oatmeal*

Bring water to a boil in a saucepan over medium heat. Remove water from heat and add the coconut milk. Stir in the oatmeal. Let stand for 2 to 3 minutes, stirring occasionally. *Serves 4*

Note: This is a quick and filling breakfast or afternoon snack that is a great pick-me-up. The coconut milk adds a touch of the good medium-chain fatty acids that are the "good" saturated fats known to boost the immune system by fighting fungi and microbes in the body.

Gluten-free	*Casein-free*	*Yeast-free*	*Egg-free*	*Soy-free*

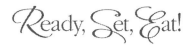

Berry Rich Breakfast Risotto

Preparation Time: 10 minutes   *Cooking Time: 45 minutes*

5   cups water
1   cup fresh or canned organic
    coconut milk*
1/2 teaspoon cinnamon*
2   teaspoons gluten-free vanilla extract*

1/4 cup beet sugar*
1   cup arborio rice
1/2 cup fresh or frozen organic
    raspberries or blueberries, rinsed

Bring the water to a boil in a medium saucepan over high heat. Pour the coconut milk, cinnamon, vanilla, sugar and 1 cup of the boiling water into a large frying pan. Stir in the rice and cook over medium-high heat, stirring constantly until the liquid is absorbed. Add the remaining water 1 cup at a time, cooking until absorbed after each addition and stirring constantly. Taste after about 45 minutes. The ideal texture of risotto is soft and silky, not mushy. Remove from the heat and fold in the berries. Serve warm. ***Serves 4***

Note: This silky, hearty dish is great as a light summer breakfast by itself. If you are a vegetarian or just wish to add some protein, vitamins B2, B complex, biotin, calcium, chromium, zinc, and good vegetable fats, add one cup of chopped organic walnuts, pecans, almonds, or sunflower seeds and serve as a light lunch or dinner. Due to the high-starch content of rice, this recipe is ideal for children or adults who wish to gain weight.

Gluten-free	*Casein-free*	*Soy-free*	*Yeast-free*

Sweet Potato Hash Browns

Preparation Time: 20 minutes   *Cooking Time: 30 minutes*

2   large sweet potatoes
1/4 cup extra-virgin olive oil

2   teaspoons organic sea salt

Peel the potatoes and submerge in a large bowl of cold water for 15 minutes; drain. Grate the potatoes with a box grater. Pat dry on a plate lined with paper towels. Heat the oil in a medium skillet over medium heat until waves form on the bottom. Fry the grated sweet potatoes in the skillet for about 5 to 6 minutes; do not stir. Flip the sweet potatoes with a spatula and cook the remaining side for 5 to 6 minutes; do not stir. Sprinkle with salt. Serve warm with gluten-free Canadian bacon or turkey sausage*. ***Serves 2***

Gluten-free	*Casein-free*	*Soy-free*	*Yeast-free*	*Nut-free*

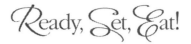

Fruit Salad with Crunchy Topping

Preparation Time: 5 minutes

1 cup fresh organic strawberries
1 cup fresh organic grapefruit sections
1 cup sliced organic banana
1 to 2 tablespoons cultured organic coconut milk* (vanilla flavored)
1/2 cup chopped organic pecans

Chop the fruits into small bite-size pieces. Place in a serving bowl and mix gently. Drizzle with the coconut milk. Sprinkle with the pecans. *Serves 4*

Tip: This easy and scrumptious fruit salad could be served with a vitamin-rich breakfast or by itself as a snack. Remember not to mix fruit with meat or protein as the acidity of the fruit will slow down the digestion of protein.

Gluten-free	Casein-free	Soy-free	Egg-free	Yeast-free

Coconut Lava

Preparation Time: 15 minutes

2 cups cultured coconut yogurt*
2 tablespoons raw sunflower seeds
2 tablespoons unsweetened sulfur-free shredded coconut
1/4 cup crunchy flax cereal*
1/4 cup miniature chocolate chips

Divide the coconut yogurt between 2 ice cream goblets or glass dessert cups. Sprinkle the yogurt with the sunflower seeds, coconut, flax cereal and chocolate chips. *Serves 2*

Note: This simple high-zinc, high-iron, moderate-sugar breakfast is done in minutes! Your brain will get a jump start with the power of one bowl of Coconut Lava!

Gluten-free	Casein-free	Yeast-free	Egg-free	Soy-free	Nut-free

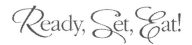

Mango Orange Shake

Preparation Time: 10 minutes   Blending Time: 1 minute

1 organic Manila mango, chopped
1 cup freshly squeezed orange juice
1 (1-inch) cube crystallized ginger, grated
1 cup ice cubes

Combine all the ingredients in an electric blender. Process until smooth. Serve immediately with breakfast or as a refreshing beverage. *Serves 4*

Note: The Manila mango has a silky texture and it is less fibrous than a regular mango. This is a favorite of children who have a sweet tooth, and it will not cause a sugar low afterward. For extra protein, you may add two tablespoons of hemp milk.

Gluten-free	*Casein-free*	*Egg-free*	*Soy-free*	*Yeast-free*	*Nut-free*

Mineral-Rich Shake

Preparation Time: 3 minutes   Blending Time: 1 minute

1/2 cup organic coconut milk*
2 cups unsweetened almond milk
   (vanilla flavored)
1/2 cup frozen organic berries
2 tablespoons brown rice
   protein powder
1 tablespoon organic blue agave nectar
1/4 cup crushed ice

Combine the coconut milk, almond milk and berries in an electric blender. Add the rice protein powder, nectar and crushed ice. Pulse a few times to mix. Blend on high speed for about 1 minute. *Serves 4*

Variation: For variety, you can use 100 percent egg white protein powder (for those not allergic to eggs) or hemp or pea protein powder instead of the brown rice protein powder. Each of the listed protein substitutions has a different nutrient composition that can be incorporated in your diet based on your individual nutritional needs.

Gluten-free	*Casein-free*	*Yeast-free*	*Egg-free*

Organic Light Agave Nectar: In some recipes where a deep flavored sweetener is needed I used certified organic agave nectar which happens to have a low glycemic index (GI) of 32, which means that it slowly absorbs in the blood stream, preventing a sugar spike. It's better for diabetics than maple sugar, which has a 54 GI. Agave nectar is sweeter than table sugar, so you can use less in any recipe that calls for sugar, honey, or maple syrup.

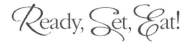
Wake-Up-Your-Brain Shake

Preparation Time: 3 minutes   Blending Time: 1 minute

2 large Haas avocados
2 cups organic coconut milk*
1/2 cup frozen organic blueberries
2 teaspoons organic blue agave nectar*

Peel and pit the avocados and place in an electric blender. Add the coconut milk, blueberries and nectar. Blend at high speed for about 1 minute. **Serves 4**

Note: This silky shake is filled with beneficial medium-chain fatty acids from coconut milk that help improve digestive health and strengthen the immune system. Avocados also contain necessary minerals like potassium, folic acid, calcium, vitamins C and K, copper, sodium, and dietary fibers.

Gluten-free	*Casein-free*	*Yeast-free*	*Egg-free*	*Nut-free*

Piña Colada Shake

Preparation Time: 10 minutes   Blending Time: 1 minute

1 cup organic coconut milk*
1 cup freshly squeezed lemon juice
1/2 cup pineapple chunks
1/2 cup ice cubes

Combine all the ingredients in an electric blender and process until smooth. Serve immediately with breakfast or as a refreshing beverage. **Serves 4**

Note: This shake has zero cholesterol and less than ten grams of fruit sugar per serving. For extra protein, you may add two tablespoons of hemp protein or 100 percent egg protein (if you're not allergic to eggs).

Gluten-free	*Casein-free*	*Egg-free*	*Soy-free*	*Yeast-free*	*Nut-free*

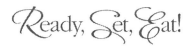

Skinny Berry Shake

Preparation Time: 5 minutes   Blending Time: 1 minute

1 cup organic strawberries
1 cup organic blueberries
Juice of 1 lemon
1 small piece fresh ginger, finely grated
$1/2$ cup ice cubes

Combine all the ingredients in an electric blender and process until smooth. Pour into 4 glasses and garnish each with a fresh mint sprig. *Serves 4*

Note: This shake has zero fat and 5 grams of fruit sugar per serving.

Gluten-free	Casein-free	Egg-free	Soy-free	Yeast-free	Nut-free

If using strawberries out of season, they're likely imported from countries that use less stringent regulations for pesticide use. Strawberries rank number 3 on the 2010 Dirty Dozen list, with 59 pesticides used on them. To avoid toxicity, buy organic and local. If unavailable, replace with kiwi or papaya.

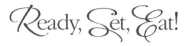

Zesty Corn Bread

Preparation Time: 15 minutes   *Cooking Time: 40 to 45 minutes*

10 ounces gluten-free fine
    yellow cornmeal
2 tablespoons brown sugar
2 teaspoons baking powder
1 teaspoon organic sea salt

1 cup gluten-free rice milk
2 eggs, or equivalent amount of
    egg substitute
2 ounces butter substitute*
2 tablespoons chopped pimentos

Preheat the oven to 400 degrees. Oil a baking pan lightly. Combine the cornmeal, brown sugar, baking powder and salt in a large bowl. Make a well in the center. Beat the rice milk, eggs and butter in a small bowl. Add to the cornmeal mixture and beat until a soft batter is formed. Fold in the pimentos. Pour the batter into the prepared pan. Bake for 40 minutes or until the corn bread tests done. Cool on a wire rack. Cut into 10 squares. **Serves 10**

Gluten-free	*Casein-free*	*Yeast-free*	*Egg-free*

Megan's Pumpkin Chocolate Chip Muffins

Preparation Time: 15 minutes   *Baking Time: 30 to 35 minutes*

1³/₄ cups certified gluten-free oat flour
¹/₂ cup beet sugar
1 teaspoon baking soda
1 teaspoon cinnamon
1 teaspoon pumpkin pie spice
¹/₈ teaspoon organic sea salt

1¹/₄ cups pumpkin purée
¹/₂ cup butter substitute*, melted
¹/₄ cup applesauce
2 tablespoons apple butter
¹/₃ cup rice milk
1 cup vegan chocolate chips*

Preheat oven to 350 degrees. Combine oat flour, sugar, baking soda, cinnamon, pumpkin pie spice and salt together. Mix the pumpkin purée, butter, applesauce, apple butter and rice milk in a large bowl. Add the dry ingredients and mix well. Stir in the chocolate chips. Fill greased muffin cups ²/₃ full. Bake for 30 to 35 minutes or until the muffins test done. **Makes 12 muffins**

Note: These naturally sweet muffins are a favorite of children around Halloween and Thanksgiving.

Gluten-free	*Casein-free*	*Nut-free*

Flaky Buttermilk Biscuits

Preparation Time: 15 to 20 minutes   *Baking Time: 10 to 12 minutes*

2   cups gluten-free all-purpose flour
2   teaspoons gluten-free baking powder
2   teaspoons baking soda (optional)
1   teaspoon beet sugar

1/2 teaspoon organic sea salt
8   tablespoons cold unsalted butter
      substitute*, cut into 1-inch cubes
3/4 cup cold buttermilk

Move an oven rack to the middle position and preheat the oven to 450 degrees. Combine the flour, baking powder, baking soda, sugar and salt in a large bowl or a food processor fitted with a steel blade. Whisk together or pulse 6 times. Use your fingertips to quickly pinch the cut up butter into the dry ingredients until the mix resembles coarse meal, or use a food processor, and drop the butter over the dry ingredients. Pulse 10 times. Stir in the buttermilk and mix with a fork until the dough forms a soft ball. If using a food processor, pour the buttermilk over the dough. Pulse 8 times. Transfer the dough to a lightly floured surface and quickly form into a ball; do not overmix. Pinch off a golf ball-size piece of dough and place on an ungreased baking sheet. Flatten with the palm of your hand to at least a 1-inch thickness. Repeat with the remaining dough. Bake immediately for 10 to 12 minutes as they need quick heat. ***Makes 12 small biscuits***

Note: These flaky biscuits are best when served warm with dairy-free butter substitute* as a side with Crispy Chicken Nuggets (page 105) or Oven-Roasted Turkey (page 108) or for breakfast with eggs or bacon. Do not substitute milk for buttermilk, as the acid in buttermilk reacts with the leavener to make the biscuit rise higher. Since most gluten-free all-purpose flours contain xanthan gum as leavener, there is no need for additional baking soda. You can double or triple this recipe and store the leftovers in an airtight container in the refrigerator for up to one week.

Gluten-free	*Yeast-free*	*Nut-free*	*Egg-free*

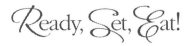

Quick and Tasty Garlic Toast

Preparation Time: 5 minutes   Cooking Time: 3 minutes

4   garlic cloves   1/2 cup butter substitute*
8   slices gluten-free white bread

Preheat the oven to 200 degrees. Cut the garlic into halves crosswise. Rub the garlic all over each bread slice. Spread a thin layer of butter on each bread slice. Place the bread butter sides up on an ungreased baking sheet. Warm for 2 to 3 minutes or until the butter has melted. *Serves 8*

Variation: You can use gluten-free whole grain bread as a wholesome alternative!

Gluten-free	*Casein-free*	*Egg-free*	*Soy-free*

Mineral-Packed Trail Mix

Preparation Time: 5 minutes

2 cups pretzels*
1/2 cup raw pumpkin seeds
1 cup carob chips
1 cup black currants
1/2 cup raw sunflower seeds

Mix all the ingredients together. Fill each of 5 small sandwich bags with 1/2 cup of the trail mix for individual snacks. *Yields 5 snack bags*

Tip: Use this every weekday as a high-zinc, high-magnesium snack that is both nutritious and delicious!

Gluten-free	*Casein-free*	*Egg-free*	*Soy-free*	*Lactose-free*

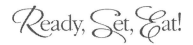

Avocado Dip

Preparation Time: 10 minutes

1 large avocado, mashed
Juice of 1 lemon
$1/3$ cup extra-virgin olive oil

1 teaspoon dried herbes de Provence
1 teaspoon organic sea salt

Combine all the ingredients in a medium bowl and mix together with a fork. Serve with your favorite vegetables such as baby carrots, celery sticks or sweet potato chips. *Serves 4 to 6*

Variation: Add $1/3$ cup raw apple cider vinegar to make a delicious creamy **Avocado Dressing** to serve on any of your favorite salads.

Gluten-free	Casein-free	Soy-free	Egg-free	Yeast-free	Nut-free

Creamy Snappy Guacamole

Preparation Time: 15 minutes

3 large Haas avocados
2 tablespoons chopped fresh
 red onion
2 tablespoons chopped fresh cilantro

2 tablespoons chopped seeded tomato
2 tablespoons lemon juice
$1/4$ teaspoon organic sea salt

Scoop the avocado into a medium bowl. Add the remaining ingredients and mash with a fork to the desired consistency. *Yields 1 1/2 cups guacamole*

Note: This Southwestern dish could be served as a starter or a snack with gluten-free corn chips or rice crackers. To encourage children to try this, ask them to help with scooping and mashing avocados, which is great sensory stimulation while learning about good fruits and vegetables.

Gluten-free	Casein-free	Yeast-free	Egg-free	Soy-free	Sugar-free

Soups, Salads, and Sides

The Recipes

- Artichoke Soup in a Flash
- Creamy Cauliflower and Broccoli Soup
- Savory Butternut Squash Soup
- Creamy Sweet Potato Soup
- Energy-Packed Bone Stock
- Red Cabbage and Onion Salad
- Chilled Cucumber and Red Onion Salad
- Endive Salad
- Jungle Salad
- Mixed Dark Green Salad
- Chicken Potato Salad
- Exotic Salad Niçoise
- Parisian Vinaigrette

- Faye's Foolproof Vinaigrette
- Almonaise (Egg-Free Mayonnaise)
- Roasted Asparagus and Cinnamon Sweet Potatoes
- Millet and Asparagus
- Faye's Green Bean Casserole
- Sweet Carrot and Pistachio Rice
- Eggplant Baba Ghanoush
- Roasted Vegetables
- Baked Spaghetti Squash
- Baked Sweet Potatoes in Syrup
- Organic Rice Macaroni and Cheese
- Quinoa Linguini Alfredo
- Almond and Cranberry Rice

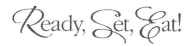

Artichoke Soup in a Flash

Preparation Time: 15 minutes   *Cooking Time: 15 minutes*

5 garlic cloves, minced
2 tablespoons extra-virgin olive oil
5 jarred or frozen small artichoke
   hearts, trimmed and chopped

Organic sea salt and pepper to taste
$^1/_2$ cup organic vegetable stock
$^1/_2$ cup water

Heat a large soup pot over medium heat. Add the garlic and drizzle with the olive oil. Cook the garlic until lightly golden, tossing or stirring occasionally. Add the artichokes, salt and pepper and stir for 1 minute. Add the stock and water. Reduce the heat to low and cook for 15 minutes. Serve with Quick and Tasty Garlic Toast (page 78). *Serves 2 to 4*

Gluten-free	*Casein-free*	*Yeast-free*	*Egg-free*	*Soy-free*

Creamy Cauliflower and Broccoli Soup

Preparation Time: 20 minutes   *Cooking Time: 20 minutes*

$^1/_2$ yellow onion, chopped
1 head of cauliflower, cut into
   4-inch pieces
1 head of broccoli, cut into
   4-inch pieces

2 tablespoons olive oil
2 cups organic chicken broth
Organic sea salt to taste
Chopped fresh thyme to taste

Sauté the onion, cauliflower and broccoli in olive oil in a large pot over medium heat until all the vegetables are lightly golden. Add the chicken broth and stir. Cover the pot, reduce the heat to low and cook for 20 minutes. Purée the soup vegetables with an immersion blender until creamy. Add salt and thyme for flavor. *Serves 6*

Note: This is a delicate, easy, and elegant soup that is bound to amaze your family and friends. You can substitute acorn squash or spaghetti squash for the cauliflower and broccoli for a fast and tasty variation.

Gluten-free	*Casein-free*	*Yeast-free*	*Soy-free*	*Egg-free*

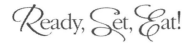

Savory Butternut Squash Soup

Preparation Time: 15 minutes   *Cooking Time: 15 minutes*

1 butternut squash, peeled and
   chopped
1/2 cup organic applesauce
1 yellow onion, chopped
2 small carrots, peeled and chopped

4 cups (1 quart) organic chicken stock
1/4 cup coconut milk*
1 pinch of organic sea salt
1 pinch of nutmeg
Juice of 1 lime

Combine the first 5 ingredients in a large soup pot and bring to a boil. Stir in the coconut milk, salt, nutmeg and lime juice. Cook for 10 minutes. Remove from the heat and blend with an immersion blender until smooth and creamy. Serve warm. ***Serves 4***

Gluten-free	*Casein-free*	*Egg-free*	*Soy-free*

Creamy Sweet Potato Soup

Preparation Time: 15 minutes   *Cooking Time: 15 minutes*

2 large sweet potatoes
1 tablespoon olive oil
2 garlic cloves, chopped

4 cups (1 quart) low-sodium
   chicken broth

Peel and cut the sweet potatoes into quarters. Sauté in the olive oil in a large soup pot over medium heat for 2 to 3 minutes or until all sides are golden. Add the garlic and sauté for 1 minute. Add the broth. Reduce the heat to medium-low and cook for about 10 minutes or until the sweet potatoes are tender. Remove from heat. Purée the sweet potatoes with an immersion blender until smooth. Serve warm. ***Serves 4***

Nutrition Scoop: This creamy sweet potato purée is chock-full of vitamins A, C, and E and is nutritionist approved and kid friendly.

Note: You could substitute butternut squash, acorn squash, or Idaho potatoes for the sweet potatoes. This is a scrumptious creamy vegetable soup on a cold winter night.

Gluten-free	*Dairy-free*	*Yeast-free*	*Egg-free*	*Nut-free*	*Lactose-free*

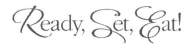

Energy-Packed Bone Stock

Preparation Time: 15 minutes   Cooking Time: 4 hours

1 organic free-range chicken, or 1 large lamb shank or
beef shank with meat, or 4 wild fish filets
2 large carrots, chopped
2 yellow onions, chopped
2 stalks celery, chopped
2 tablespoons lemon juice or vinegar
1 pinch of herbes de Provence
2 teaspoons organic sea salt
1/2 teaspoon black pepper

Rinse the chicken. Place in a large soup pot. Add the carrots, onions, celery and lemon juice. Season with the herbes de Provence, salt and pepper. Cover with water. Cook, covered, over medium-low heat for 4 hours. Skim off any fat that may have risen to the surface. Strain the stock into a large bowl, discarding the solids. Serve in soup bowls or use as the base for Creamy Sweet Potato Soup (page 82). ***Serves 4***

Gluten-free	*Casein-free*	*Yeast-free*	*Soy-free*	*Low-Oxalate*

Sea Salt: I use a blend of Himalayan pink salt, Bolivian rose salt, Hawaiian alaea sea salt, and Chinese sea salt from Ming Dynasty Saltworks. Sea salt, though more expensive than table salt, is well worth the extra investment in your health, as its platinum group elements support continuous energy release, immediate hydration and high electrolyte levels. It is great for athletes, active children, and all people who seek its health benefits and taste. Other sources, like Celtic sea salt, are also acceptable.

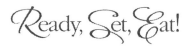

Red Cabbage and Onion Salad

Preparation Time: 10 minutes

3 cups shredded red cabbage
1 cup finely chopped red onion
1/4 cup salted raw sunflower seeds
1/2 cup extra-virgin olive oil

1/4 cup balsamic vinegar
1 teaspoon herbes de Provence*
1/2 teaspoon organic sea salt
1/4 teaspoon freshly ground black pepper

Rinse and drain the cabbage. Combine with the onion and sunflower seeds in a large bowl. Mix the olive oil, balsamic vinegar, herbes de Provence, salt and pepper in a small bowl. Pour the dressing onto the salad mixture and toss to coat evenly. *Serves 6 to 8*

Photo for this recipe on page 53.

Gluten-free   *Casein-free*

Chilled Cucumber and Red Onion Salad

Preparation Time: 10 minutes   *Chilling Time: 2 hours or more*

1 large cucumber
1/8 to 1/4 red onion
1 plum tomato, sliced, or 3 or 4 cherry tomatoes, halved
Parisian Vinaigrette (page 88)
1 tablespoon chopped fresh dill weed or mint

Peel the cucumber, if desired, and slice thinly. Slice the red onion. Combine the cucumber, onion and tomato in a bowl. Drizzle with the desired amount of dressing and toss well. Sprinkle with the dill weed. Cover the bowl and chill in the refrigerator for 2 hours or more before serving. *Serves 2*

Note: Recipe can be doubled or tripled.

Gluten-free   *Casein-free*

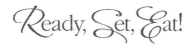

Endive Salad

Preparation Time: 15 minutes

4   avocados, peeled
4   heads endive
2   Granny Smith apples

1/4 cup dried cranberries
Vinaigrette

Cut the avocados into chunks. Place in a large salad bowl. Clean the endive leaves thoroughly; pat dry and cut into slices. Mix with the avocados. Cut the apples into 2-inch chunks and add to salad bowl with the dried cranberries. Drizzle the desired amount of vinaigrette over salad, toss and serve. *Serves 4*

Gluten-free	*Casein-free*	*Soy-free*	*Yeast-free*

Jungle Salad

Preparation Time: 20 minutes

1   head Boston lettuce, torn
3   or 4 baby carrots, julienned

8   cherry tomatoes
Sweet-and-Sour Dressing (below)

Combine the lettuce, carrots and cherry tomatoes in a salad bowl and toss lightly. Add the desired amount of dressing and toss to mix. *Serves 4*

Sweet-and-Sour Dressing

1/2 cup extra-virgin olive oil
1/4 cup red wine vinegar
1   tablespoon balsamic vinegar
1   teaspoon sugar

1   teaspoon Dijon mustard
Garlic powder, organic sea salt and
    pepper to taste

Combine the olive oil and remaining ingredients in a small jar. Shake to mix well and pour over salad. *Serves 4*

Gluten-free	*Casein-free*	*Yeast-free*	*Soy-free*

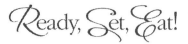
Mixed Dark Green Salad

Preparation Time: 10 minutes

16 ounces mixed organic salad greens
1 Haas avocado
1/2 small red onion
Lemon Vinaigrette (below)

Place the salad greens in a bowl. Cut the avocado 1-inch slices. Cut the onion into thin slices. Arrange the slices over the salad greens. Drizzle with Lemon Vinaigrette and garnish with chopped chives. *Serves 4*

Lemon Vinaigrette

1/2 cup extra-virgin olive oil
1 teaspoon prepared mustard
1/2 teaspoon beet sugar
Juice and zest of 1/2 lemon
Organic sea salt and pepper to taste

Combine all the ingredients in a jar with a tight-fitting lid. Cover tightly and shake vigorously.

Gluten-free   *Casein-free*   *Yeast-free*   *Soy-free*

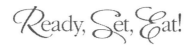

Chicken Potato Salad

Preparation Time: 15 minutes   Cooking Time: 10 minutes

4	cups (about) water	3	dill pickles, chopped
3	Idaho potatoes	3	tablespoons mayonnaise
2	cups frozen green peas		Organic sea salt to taste
1	roasted 2-pound rotisserie chicken		

Bring the water to a boil in a large pot. Add the unpeeled potatoes and cook for about 5 minutes or until fork-tender. Remove potatoes from the pot and let cool. Peel the potatoes and chop into 2-inch pieces. Place in a large glass mixing bowl. Steam the green peas for 2 minutes. Cut the chicken into 3- to 4-inch pieces. Chop the pickles into bite-size piece. Add the peas, chicken and pickles to the potatoes in the bowl. Add the mayonnaise and salt and mix lightly. *Serves 4*

Note: This is a versatile potato salad that could be kept in the refrigerator for up to three days. You can wrap it in a brown rice tortilla as a hearty lunch or enjoy a smaller portion with some rice or corn chips as a snack.

Gluten-free   Yeast-free

Exotic Salad Niçoise

Preparation Time: 15 minutes

1	head red-tip lettuce, torn	1	(4-ounce) can sardines in oil, drained
2	hard-cooked free-range eggs, chopped	10	to 15 kalamata olives
1	(6-ounce) can white tuna in water, drained	1	or 2 slivers of red onion
		6	cherry tomatoes
			Vinaigrette

Combine the lettuce, eggs, tuna, sardines, olives, onion and tomatoes in a large bowl. Drizzle with the desired amount of dressing and toss lightly. *Serves 4 to 6*

Photo for this recipe on page 54.

Gluten-free   Casein-free   Yeast-free   Soy-free

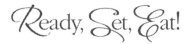

Parisian Vinaigrette

Preparation Time: 5 minutes

2/3 cup olive oil or flax oil
1 tablespoon Dijon mustard
1/4 cup balsamic vinegar or lemon juice
1 garlic clove, minced
1/4 cup water
Gluten-free dried herbes de Provence to taste

Combine all the ingredients into a jar with a tight-fitting lid. Seal tightly and shake vigorously to mix well. *Serves 6*

Gluten-free　　　*Casein-free*

Faye's Foolproof Vinaigrette

Preparation Time: 5 minutes

2 teaspoons beet sugar
1 tablespoon Dijon mustard
1/2 cup extra-virgin olive oil
1/4 cup balsamic vinegar
1 pinch of organic sea salt
Freshly ground pepper to taste

Mix the sugar and Dijon mustard in a bowl. Add the olive oil gradually, whisking constantly. Add the vinegar and season with the salt and pepper. *Makes 3/4 cup*

Gluten-free　　　*Casein-free*　　　*Yeast-free*　　　*Egg-free*

Almonaise
(Egg-Free Mayonnaise)

Preparation Time: 5 minutes

Water for boiling
1/2 cup unblanched almonds
1/2 cup (or more) purified water
1 small sliver of garlic
1/2 teaspoon organic sea salt
2 to 3 tablespoons freshly squeezed lemon juice
Freshly ground pepper to taste
2 to 3 cups olive oil

Bring water to a boil in a small saucepan. Drop the almonds in the boiling water for just 1 minute. Remove from heat and drain. Place the almonds in a bowl of ice water; the almonds' peels should separate. Remove the peels by gently pinching the almonds. Combine the almonds and purified water in a blender and blend on high speed until thick. If the mixture is difficult to blend, add 1 to 2 tablespoons water until blade moves freely. Add the garlic, salt, lemon juice and pepper. Blend for 30 seconds. Remove the center plug from the top of the blender pitcher and slowly drizzle the olive oil into the almond mixture with the blender running. The blade will turn more and more freely as you blend. When the olive oil begins to sit in a bubble on top of the almond mixture, turn off the blender. Continue to add the remaining olive oil in a thin stream, mixing gently with a spoon. This will force more olive oil into the mixture and make a thicker product. Store in a covered glass container in the refrigerator for up to 1 week. ***Makes 3 cups***

Note: If you blend all the ingredients together at once, the almonaise will be bitter.

Gluten-free	*Casein-free*	*Yeast-free*	*Egg-free*

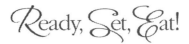

Roasted Asparagus and Cinnamon Sweet Potatoes

Preparation Time: 10 minutes   Cooking Time: 30 minutes

1 pound fresh organic asparagus
2 large sweet potatoes, cut into halves horizontally
¼ cup olive oil
Coarse organic sea salt to taste
Cinnamon to taste

Preheat the oven to 300 degrees. Boil the sweet potatoes in water to cover in a saucepan for 10 minutes or until fork-tender. Snap off the thick, woody ends of the asparagus spears and discard. Remove the sweet potatoes from the pan and pat dry. Arrange the sweet potatoes and asparagus on a baking sheet. Drizzle with the olive oil and sprinkle with salt. Sprinkle cinnamon over the sweet potatoes. Roast on the the middle oven rack for 25 to 30 minutes. **Serves 4**

Note: This is an easy and elegant side dish that can accompany any entrée.

Gluten-free	Casein-free	Egg-free	Soy-free	Yeast-free

Millet and Asparagus

Preparation Time: 15 minutes   Cooking Time: 15 minutes

3 cups vegetable stock
1 cup millet grain
½ teaspoon organic sea salt
1½ cups chopped fresh asparagus tips
1 tablespoon butter substitute*
½ bunch basil, finely chopped
Pepper to taste
Juice of 1 lemon

Bring the stock to a boil in a saucepan. Place the millet in a dry pan or pot over low heat. Toast until the millet emits a nutty fragrance, stirring constantly. Add the boiling stock and salt to the millet. Add the asparagus tips and return to a boil. Cover the pan and reduce the heat. Simmer for 20 to 25 minutes or until all the liquid is absorbed. Add the butter. Let stand, covered, for 5 minutes. Add the basil, pepper and lemon juice and toss lightly to mix. **Serves 4**

Gluten-free	Casein-free	Soy-free	Yeast-free

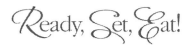

Faye's Green Bean Casserole

Preparation Time: 15 minutes   Baking Time: 45 minutes

1 tablespoon olive oil
2 cups butter substitute
2 cups rice flour
4 to 5 cups free-range organic chicken broth
1 (24-ounce) package frozen green beans
Organic sea salt and pepper to taste
8 ounces sliced roasted almonds

Preheat the oven to 350 degrees. Grease a rectangular baking dish with the olive oil. Melt the butter in a saucepan over medium heat. Add the rice flour and whisk until smooth. Add 4 cups of the broth gradually, whisking constantly until the mixture is light and creamy and adding additional broth if needed to reach the desired consistency. Taste and season with salt and pepper, if desired. Arrange half the green beans in the prepared dish. Pour half the sauce over the green beans. Repeat the layering process. Sprinkle with the almonds. Bake for 45 minutes. *Serves 6*

Variation: For casein-tolerant individuals, substitute 2 cups half-and-half for 1 cup of the butter substitute.

Photo for this recipe on page 51.

Gluten-free   Casein-free

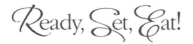

Sweet Carrot and Pistachio Rice

Preparation Time: 10 minutes   Cooking Time: 20 minutes

4   cups water
1   cup long-grain basmati rice, rinsed
1   pinch of organic sea salt
3   tablespoons vegetable oil

2   large organic carrots, peeled
    and julienned
1/4 cup chopped roasted pistachios

Combine the water, rice, salt and 2 tablespoons of the oil in a rice cooker. Cook using the manufacturer's directions. Sauté the carrots in the remaining 1 tablespoon oil in a skillet over low heat for a few minutes or until shiny. Top the rice with the carrots and pistachios and serve warm. *Serves 4 to 6*

Note: This is a very simple and snappy summer side dish that would complement either beef or chicken kabobs. You can whip this up with the help of a rice cooker in about 30 minutes. It can be doubled to serve on two separate weeknights.

Gluten-free	*Casein-free*	*Yeast-free*	*Soy-free*	*Egg-free*

Eggplant Baba Ghanoush

Preparation Time: 15 minutes   Cooking Time: 20 minutes

2   eggplant
Organic sea salt to taste
1   yellow onion, finely chopped

2   to 3 tablespoons olive oil
1   teaspoon cumin
Pepper to taste

Peel the eggplant and cut crosswise into 2-inch slices. Salt both sides generously and place in a colander. Let the slices sweat until droplets form on the eggplant. Rinse off the salt and pat the eggplant slices dry on a large tray. Sauté the onion in 1 to 2 teaspoons of the olive oil in a large skillet until golden. Remove the onion to a small bowl. Pour the remaining olive oil into a skillet. Fry the eggplant slices in the oil over low heat on both sides until golden. Combine the eggplant slices and the onion in a serving bowl. Mash with a fork. Season with cumin, salt and pepper. Garnish with a mint sprig. *Serves 4*

Gluten-free	*Casein-free*	*Egg-free*	*Nut-free*	*Lactose-free*	*Yeast-free*

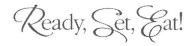

Roasted Vegetables

Preparation Time: 15 minutes   *Cooking Time: 30 minutes*

2 red bell peppers	¹/₂ red onion, sliced
2 yellow bell peppers	¹/₄ cup olive oil
1 pound fresh organic asparagus	Coarse organic sea salt

Preheat the oven to 300 degrees. Remove the skin if using non-organic vegetables. Cut each pepper into 4 strips. Place inside up on a large baking sheet. Arrange the asparagus and onion on the baking sheet. Drizzle the vegetables with the olive oil and sprinkle with salt. Roast for about 30 minutes. *Serves 6 to 8*

Note: A simple and quick side dish that accompanies any entrée is roasted vegetables.

Gluten-free	*Casein-free*	*Egg-free*	*Soy-free*	*Yeast-free*

Baked Spaghetti Squash

Preparation Time: 15 minutes   *Cooking Time: 20 minutes*

2 spaghetti squash
Butter substitute*
Herbs or salsa to taste

Preheat the oven to 375 degrees. Make deep pierces into the skin of the squash in several places using a long-tined fork; place in a baking dish. Bake for about 30 minutes or until the skin is soft to the touch. Cool for 10 minutes. Cut each into halves lengthwise. Use a spoon to remove the seeds from the center of the squash. Use two forks to fluff up the squash until you have spaghetti-like strands. Transfer the strands to a serving plate and top with butter and herbs or salsa. *Serves 4*

Gluten-free	*Casein-free*	*Yeast-free*	*Soy-free*

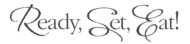
Baked Sweet Potatoes in Syrup

Preparation Time: 5 minutes   Cooking Time: 1 hour

4   large sweet potatoes
1/4 cup apple cider
1/4 cup packed brown sugar
1/4 teaspoon cinnamon

1/8 teaspoon ground nutmeg
2   tablespoons butter substitute*
2   tablespoons grated orange zest

Preheat the oven to 350 degrees. Boil the sweet potatoes in water to cover in a large
pot for 20 to 30 minutes or until almost fork-tender; drain. Peel the potatoes and cut
into 1/4-inch slices. Layer into a shallow round baking dish. Pour the cider into a small
saucepan over medium heat and reduce by half. Stir in the brown sugar, cinnamon
and nutmeg. Remove from the heat and add the butter and orange zest. Pour over the
potatoes. Bake, covered, for about 30 minutes. *Serves 8*

Gluten-free	*Casein-free*	*Egg-free*	*Yeast-free*

Organic Rice Macaroni and Cheese

Preparation Time: 5 minutes   Cooking Time: 15 minutes

8   cups water
2   teaspoons organic sea salt
3   tablespoons olive oil
2   cups gluten-free elbow rice macaroni*

2   teaspoons cornstarch
3/4 cup rice milk
1   cup shredded vegan Cheddar cheese*

Bring the water to a boil in a large saucepan over medium heat. Add the salt, 1 tablespoon
of the olive oil and the pasta to the water. Cook for about 8 minutes or until the pasta is
al dente; drain. Heat the remaining 2 tablespoons olive oil in a saucepan over low heat.
Whisk the cornstarch into the rice milk in a small bowl. Add to the heated olive oil. Cook
until the mixture begins to thicken, whisking constantly. Add the cheese and cook until the
cheese is melted and the mixture is smooth. You may also use an immersion blender to
blend until smooth. Add the pasta and stir until coated. Serve warm. *Serves 8*

Photo for this recipe on page 51.

Gluten-free	*Casein-free*	*Yeast-free*

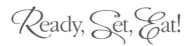

Quinoa Linguini Alfredo

Preparation Time: 15 minutes   Cooking Time: 15 minutes

4 cups water
8 ounces quinoa linguini
1 pinch of organic sea salt
1/2 cup extra-virgin olive oil
1/2 cup butter substitute*
1/2 cup mozzarella-flavor cheese substitute*
3 tablespoons chopped fresh basil

Bring the water to a boil in a large pot. Add the linguini, salt and 1 tablespoon of the olive oil. Return to a boil and cover. Cook for about 6 minutes, stirring once to prevent sticking; do not overcook. Drain the linguini. Heat the butter, cheese substitute and basil in a medium saucepan over low heat until the cheese substitute and butter have melted, stirring constantly. Spoon the linguini into a bowl. Drizzle with the remaining olive oil and serve warm. *Serves 4*

Note: This is a high-protein dish that is based on an ancient South American grain, quinoa. Chicken Parmesan (page 105) will nicely complement this side dish.

Gluten-free	Casein-free	Yeast-free	Egg-free

Almond and Cranberry Rice

Preparation Time: 5 minutes   Cooking Time: 20 minutes

2 cups long grain basmati and
    wild rice blend, rinsed
1/2 teaspoon ground saffron
2 tablespoons hot water

1 pinch of organic sea salt
1 tablespoon vegetable oil
1/4 cup slivered roasted almonds
1/4 cup dried cranberries

Pour the rice into a rice cooker with enough water to cover by 1 inch. Dissolve the saffron in the hot water. Add the saffron, salt and oil to the rice. Cook using the manufacturer's directions. Top with the almonds and cranberries and serve warm. *Serves 6*

Photo for this recipe on page 50.

Gluten-free	Casein-free	Soy-free	Egg-free	Yeast-free

Ready, Set, Eat!

Beef, Pork, Poultry, Seafood, and Meatless Mains

The Recipes

- Scrumptious Beef Kabobs
- Veggie Burger Burritos
- Italian Meatballs
- Beef Roast with Brussels Sprouts and Baby Carrots
- Juicy Hamburgers
- Roasted Pork Tenderloin with Mango-Ginger Chutney
- Miniature Sausage Pizzas
- Barbecue-Roasted Chicken Wings and Drumsticks
- Corn Tortilla Fajitas
- Lemon Olive Chicken
- Saffron Chicken Kabobs
- Crispy Chicken Parmesan
- Crispy Chicken Nuggets
- Lip-Smacking Barbecue Chicken Pizza
- Chicken Pot Pie
- Oven-Roasted Turkey
- Cod with Spinach and Tomatoes
- Oven-Roasted Halibut
- Crispy Salmon Nuggets
- Light Cheese Enchiladas
- Vegetable Lasagna
- Manicotti
- Hearty Vegetarian Tacos
- Pasta Primavera with Vegetables
- Baked Ziti

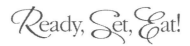

Scrumptious Beef Kabobs

Preparation Time: 20 minutes plus 1 hour marinating   Cooking Time: 5 to 6 minutes

1 (1-pound) sirloin or filet mignon steak, cut into 3 pieces
2 zucchini, cut into 3-inch slices diagonally
1 yellow onion, cut into 4 pieces
1 red bell pepper, cut into 2-inch pieces
Marinade (below)

Place the meat and vegetables in a sealable plastic bag with the Marinade. Seal the bag and turn to coat. Marinate in the refrigerator for 1 hour. Place 12 (6-inch) wooden skewers in water to cover and let soak for 1 hour. Drain the marinade and thread the meat and vegetables onto the skewers. Place the skewers on the hot grill. Grill for 2 to 3 minutes per side. *Serves 4 (3 kabobs per serving)*

Marinade

1 teaspoon minced garlic
1/2 cup wheat-free tamari sauce
1/4 cup peanut oil
1/4 teaspoon cayenne pepper
1 tablespoon lime juice
Organic sea salt and ground black pepper to taste

Mix the marinade ingredients in a bowl.

Tip: For a complete meal, serve this dish with flavored saffron rice. This makes a great summer lunch or dinner, especially when you enjoy it outdoors with your family.

Gluten-free	*Casein-free*	*Yeast-free*

According to a recent USDA Inspector General report, while beef muscle is typically clean, beef fat can contain as many as ten different pesticides.

Veggie Burger Burritos

Preparation Time: 5 minutes   Cooking Time: 15 minutes

2 pounds choice lean ground beef
1/2 yellow onion, grated
1 large carrot, grated
1 zucchini, grated
1 teaspoon cumin
1 tablespoon organic sea salt
1 teaspoon ground pepper
1 to 2 tablespoons extra-virgin olive oil
4 to 6 brown rice tortillas* or 100% corn tortillas
4 to 6 sprigs of parsley

Combine the ground beef, grated vegetables and seasonings in a large mixing bowl and mix well. Divide into equal portions and shape into oblong patties. Heat the olive oil in a large nonstick skillet over medium heat. Cook the patties for about 7 to 8 minutes on each side or to an internal temperature of 160 degrees. Place the patties on a plate lined with paper towels to drain. Place the brown rice tortillas on a flat surface. Place a patty about 2 inches away from the edge of a tortilla and roll up the tortilla to enclose the patty. Place seam side down back into the skillet to keep warm and repeat with the remaining patties and tortillas. Top each burrito with a parsley sprig and serve. ***Serves 4 to 6***

Note: This is a perfect recipe for picky eaters, as you can hide a few servings of vegetables in the burrito. This has served particularly well for those with sensory processing deficits and/or an aversion to the texture or taste of vegetables.

Gluten-free   Casein-free   Yeast-free

Italian Meatballs

Preparation Time: 20 minutes   *Cooking Time: 30 minutes*

1/2 cup minced red onion
1 tablespoon extra-virgin olive oil
1 garlic clove, chopped
1 pound ground beef
1 free-range egg
2 tablespoons tomato sauce
1 pinch of organic sea salt
1 pinch of freshly ground pepper

3 tablespoons mozzarella-flavored dairy-free gluten-free cheese
2 tablespoons gluten-free bread crumbs
1 tablespoon extra-virgin olive oil
2 tablespoons gluten-free tamari sauce
2 teaspoons apple cider vinegar
2 tablespoons gluten-free ketchup

Sauté the onion in 1 tablespoon olive oil in a large saucepan for 3 minutes. Add the garlic and cook for 3 minutes longer or until golden. Remove the onion and garlic to a mixing bowl using a slotted spoon. Set the saucepan aside. Add the ground beef, egg, tomato sauce, salt, pepper, cheese and bread crumbs to the onion mixture. Mix well and shape into golf ball-size balls. Heat the remaining 1 tablespoon olive oil in the saucepan over medium heat. Add the meatballs and cook for 5 to 6 minutes on each side; cover and keep warm. Blend the tamari sauce, vinegar and ketchup in a small bowl and drizzle over the meatballs, stirring gently to mix. *Serves 4*

Note: These are delicious on spaghetti. Just cook brown rice spaghetti* as direct on the package, adding a pinch of organic sea salt and 1 tablespoon of olive oil. Cook for 6 to 7 minutes or until tender but not mushy; drain well.

Gluten-free	*Casein-free*	*Soy-free*	*Yeast-free*

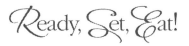

Beef Roast with Brussels Sprouts and Baby Carrots

Preparation Time: 30 minutes   *Cooking Time: 3 hours*

1 (2-pound) chuck roast	8 ounces shallots
10 garlic cloves	16 to 18 baby carrots
2 to 3 tablespoons extra-virgin olive oil	8 ounces brussels sprouts
Organic sea salt and pepper to taste	1 cup beef stock* or water
Chopped fresh rosemary to taste	

Preheat the oven to 325 degrees. Rinse the roast with water. Cut 10 slits in the roast and fill each with one of the garlic cloves. Place the roast in a Dutch oven greased with the olive oil. Cook the roast over high heat for 3 to 4 minutes on each side. Sprinkle the roast with salt, pepper and rosemary. Place the vegetables around the roast. Add the broth and place on the middle oven rack. Roast, uncovered, for 1¹/₂ hours. Turn the roast over, cover, and reduce the temperature to 250 degrees. Roast for 1¹/₂ hours longer. Place the roast and vegetables on a serving dish and pour the juices from the Dutch oven over the roast. Garnish with fresh rosemary sprigs. *Serves 8*

Note: For the greatest flavor, you need to cook this dish slow and low. It is best done on a weekend three hours prior to mealtime. Believe it, this one is worth the wait!

Photo for this recipe on page 49.

Gluten-free	*Casein-free*	*Soy-free*	*Egg-free*	*Yeast-free*	*Low-Oxalate*

Juicy Hamburgers

Preparation Time: 10 minutes   *Cooking Time: 10 minutes*

2 pounds choice lean ground beef	1 teaspoon ground pepper
¹/₂ yellow onion, grated	1 to 2 tablespoons extra-virgin olive oil
1 teaspoon ground cumin	4 to 6 gluten-free buns*
1 tablespoon organic sea salt	

Mix the ground beef, onion and seasonings together in a large mixing bowl. Shape into patties. Heat the olive oil in a large nonstick skillet over medium heat. Add the patties and cook for about 7 to 8 minutes on each side or to an internal temperature of 160 degrees. Place the patties on a plate lined with paper towels to drain. Serve the burgers on the buns. *Serves 4 to 6*

Gluten-free	*Casein-free*	*Yeast-free*

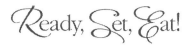

Roasted Pork Tenderloin with Mango-Ginger Chutney

Preparation Time: 10 minutes   Cooking Time: 1¹/₂ hours

1 (12-ounce) pork tenderloin, trimmed
¹/₂ cup Mango-Ginger Chutney (below)
¹/₄ cup extra-virgin olive oil

Preheat the oven to 350 degrees. Place the tenderloin in a sealable plastic bag with half the Mango-Ginger Chutney. Marinate in the refrigerator for about 1 hour. Remove the tenderloin from the bag and transfer to a roasting pan. Discard the marinade. Rub the tenderloin with the olive oil and the remaining Mango-Ginger Chutney. Roast for 1 to 1¹/₂ hours. Let stand for 15 minutes before slicing. **Serves 6**

Mango-Ginger Chutney

3 firm mangoes, chopped
¹/₂ cup apple cider vinegar
¹/₂ cup organic light brown sugar
1 (1-inch) piece fresh ginger, peeled and finely chopped
1 teaspoon organic sea salt
¹/₂ teaspoon cayenne pepper
¹/₂ teaspoon freshly ground black pepper

Bring all the ingredients to a boil in a medium saucepan over medium heat. Reduce the heat to low and simmer for 20 minutes, stirring constantly. Remove from heat and cool before serving. You can double this recipe and keep half in an airtight container in the refrigerator for later use.

Tip: For an excellent accompaniment to the roasted pork, place two cut zucchini and two carrots on an oiled baking sheet. Season lightly with salt. Roast at 350 degrees for 30 minutes.

Photo for this recipe on page 50.

Gluten-free	*Casein-free*	*Egg-free*	*Yeast-free*

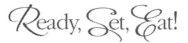

Miniature Sausage Pizzas

Preparation Time: 5 minutes   Cooking Time: 12 minutes

8 ounces gluten-free tomato sauce*
2 (8-inch) gluten-free frozen pizza crusts*
1 (8-ounce) package dairy-free gluten-free
mozzarella-flavored cheese* (or rice cheese)
4 gluten-free sausage links*, sliced and cooked

Preheat the oven to 450 degrees. Spread the tomato sauce on the pizza crusts. Sprinkle with the cheese and then top with the sausage. Bake for 10 to 12 minutes or until the cheese softens. *Serves 4*

Photo for this recipe on page 53.

Gluten-free   Casein-free

Barbecue-Roasted
Chicken Wings and Drumsticks

Preparation Time: 10 minutes   Cooking Time: 35 to 40 minutes

3 tablespoons extra-virgin olive oil
2 pounds free-range chicken wings and drumsticks
1 cup Barbecue Sauce (below)

Preheat the oven to 450 degrees. Heat the olive oil in a large ovenproof skillet. Add the chicken and sear for 3 minutes per side. Drizzle the Barbecue Sauce over the chicken and place on the middle oven rack. Bake for about 40 minutes, turning the chicken pieces over once halfway through the baking time. *Serves 4 to 6*

Barbecue Sauce

1/2 cup gluten-free ketchup*
1/4 cup gluten-free Worcestershire sauce*
1   tablespoon pure organic blue
    agave nectar*

1   tablespoon balsamic vinegar
1   teaspoon organic sea salt
3/4 cup water

Combine all the ingredients in a saucepan. Bring to a simmer over medium heat, stirring frequently.

Warning: *Sauce ingredients vary according to product availability. We do not make any guarantees as to safety of these sauce ingredients for people with food allergies or sensitivities and intolerances.

Gluten-free   Casein-free   Yeast-free

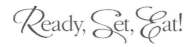
Corn Tortilla Fajitas

Preparation Time: 10 minutes   Cooking Time: 10 minutes

1 pound beef flank or boneless, skinless chicken tenders
1 tablespoon gluten-free fajita seasoning*
$^1/_2$ yellow onion
1 tablespoon extra-virgin olive oil
4 medium gluten-free corn tortillas

Cut the beef crosswise into 1-inch strips. Season with the fajita seasoning and set aside. Slice the onion crosswise into large $^1/_2$-inch rings. Sauté the onion with the beef in the olive oil in a large nonstick skillet until the beef is cooked through. (Use a meat thermometer to check doneness.) Warm the tortillas in a toaster oven for 30 seconds when ready to serve the fajitas. Scoop the meat filling into the tortillas and roll up. Garnish with fresh cilantro. *Serves 4*

Optional: You can serve this snappy, tasty dish with guacamole, chopped tomato salsa, or both. For those who are not soy-allergic, you may use soy sour cream, which is dairy-free.

Gluten-free	*Casein-free*	*Soy-free*	*Egg-free*	*Yeast-free*

Beware that chicken fat is more contaminated with pesticides than any other part of the chicken. Avoid using thigh meat, as it is the highest in fat. If making a chicken leg recipe, use free-range, pesticide-free chicken legs.

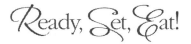

Lemon Olive Chicken

Preparation Time: 15 minutes   Cooking Time: 45 minutes

2 pounds boneless skinless chicken breasts
1¹/₂ tablespoons olive oil
4 garlic cloves, smashed
Zest of 2 lemons, cut into thin strips
Organic sea salt and pepper to taste
1 (15-ounce) can black olives, drained
1¹/₂ tablespoons chicken stock

Preheat the oven to 375 degrees. Rinse the chicken and pat dry. Arrange in a shallow baking pan. Top with the olive oil, garlic and lemon zest. Sprinkle with salt and pepper. Place the olives around the chicken and pour the stock into the pan. Bake for 45 minutes. **Serves 8**

Gluten-free	Casein-free	Yeast-free	Soy-free	Egg-free

Saffron Chicken Kabobs

Preparation Time: 40 to 45 minutes   Cooking Time: 6 minutes

1 tablespoon saffron
¹/₄ cup hot water
1 tablespoon lime juice
¹/₄ cup olive oil
Organic sea salt and pepper to taste
1 pound boneless skinless chicken breasts, cut into 1-inch pieces
10 cherry tomatoes, cut into halves

Place 6-inch wooden skewers in warm water to cover for about 30 minutes. Dissolve the saffron in the hot water. Mix the saffron water, lime juice, olive oil, salt and pepper in a small bowl. Thread the chicken and tomatos alternately onto the skewers. Brush the skewers with the saffron mixture and place on a hot grill. Grill for 2 to 3 minutes on each side, turning once. Serve warm. **Serves 4**

Gluten-free	Casein-free	Yeast-free	Egg-free

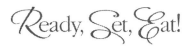

Crispy Chicken Parmesan

Preparation Time: 15 minutes   *Cooking Time: 8 to 15 minutes*

2   large boneless skinless
    chicken breasts
1/4 cup olive oil
1   cup gluten-free plain rice milk
1   cup Gluten-Free Flour Blend
    (page 67)

1   pinch of gluten-free herbes
    de Provence*
1   pinch of organic sea salt

Cut each chicken breast horizontally into 2 thin halves. Place a sheet of plastic wrap over the chicken and beat with a mallet until about 1 inch thick. Heat the olive oil in a large skillet over medium heat. Pour the milk into a wide bowl. Pour the flour onto a plate. Dip the chicken in the milk and then coat on both sides with the flour. Place the chicken in the hot oil and cook for about 4 minutes on each side. Sprinkle the chicken with the herbes de Provence and salt and serve warm. *Serves 4*

Note: If you are not allergic to eggs, replace the milk substitute with 2 beaten eggs. This will be a complete entrée if served with Quinoa Linguini Alfredo (page 95).

Gluten-free	Casein-free	Yeast-free	Soy-free	Egg-free

Crispy Chicken Nuggets

Preparation Time: 10 minutes   *Cooking Time: 20 minutes*

1 cup gluten-free Rice Chex cereal
2 teaspoons organic sea salt
1/2 teaspoon ground cumin
1 pound chicken tenders, cut into 3-inch pieces
1/2 cup butter substitute*, melted
1/4 cup extra-virgin olive oil

Heat the oven to 425 degrees. Crush the cereal in a small bowl. Mix in the salt and cumin. Dip the chicken pieces in the melted butter and then roll in the cereal mixture until evenly coated. Place the chicken on a baking sheet brushed with the olive oil. Bake for 15 to 20 minutes on the middle oven rack or until the internal temperature reaches 160 degrees. *Serves 4*

Tip: These nuggets can be baked in advance and reheated at 350 degrees for 10 minutes.

Gluten-free	Casein-free	Yeast-free

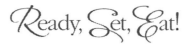

Lip-Smacking Barbecue Chicken Pizza

Preparation Time: 15 minutes   Baking Time: 15 minutes

1 yellow onion, chopped
1 tablespoon extra-virgin olive oil
1 pound chicken thighs
Organic sea salt to taste
Barbecue Sauce (below)
2 (8-inch) frozen gluten-free pizza crusts*
4 ounces dairy-free mozzarella cheese, shredded

Preheat the oven to 450 degrees. Sauté the onion in the olive oil in a large skillet over medium heat for 2 to 3 minutes or until golden. Add the chicken and salt to the skillet and cook for about 8 minutes on each side or until the chicken pulls apart from the bone. Spread Barbecue Sauce on the crusts. Layer the chicken over the sauce and sprinkle the cheese on top. Bake for 10 to 15 minutes or until the cheese softens. *Serves 4*

Barbecue Sauce

¹/₂ cup gluten-free ketchup*
¹/₂ cup gluten-free Worcestershire sauce*
1 tablespoon pure organic blue agave nectar*
1 tablespoon balsamic vinegar
1 teaspoon organic sea salt
³/₄ cup water

Combine the ketchup, Worcestershire sauce, syrup, vinegar, salt and water in a saucepan and mix well. Bring to a simmer over medium heat.

Note: This delicious pizza is unusually tasty and elegant and soon will become your household's favorite just like it did mine! Substitute chicken tenders for thighs to make a lower fat version.

Gluten-free

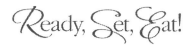

Chicken Pot Pie

Preparation Time: 30 minutes   *Cooking Time: 45 minutes*

Pastry

1   free-range egg
1¹/₄ cups Gluten-Free Flour Mix
    (page 124)
¹/₂ teaspoon xanthan gum

¹/₄ teaspoon organic sea salt
6   tablespoons cold butter
2   to 3 tablespoons cold water

Beat the egg in a small bowl and reserve 2 tablespoons for brushing the crust. Mix the dry ingredients in a large bowl. Cut in the butter until crumbly. Add the remaining egg and enough water to form a sticky dough. Shape into a ball and place between 2 sheets of waxed paper. Flatten the dough with a rolling pin to a 1-inch thickness. Wrap and refrigerate until ready to use.

Filling

2   shallots, or 1 yellow onion
4   carrots
3   stalks celery with leaves
1   whole rotisserie chicken
4   cups (or more) organic chicken stock
1   cup frozen peas
2   teaspoons organic sea salt

5   tablespoons olive oil or
    butter substitute*
¹/₂ cup gluten-free flour
¹/₃ cup coarsely chopped fresh parsley
1   teaspoon fresh tarragon, or
    ¹/₂ teaspoon dried tarragon
Pastry (above)

Preheat the oven to 425 degrees. Slice the shallots, carrots and celery into ¹/₄-inch slices diagonally. Combine with the chicken, stock, peas and salt in large stockpot. Add additional stock if needed to cover the chicken. Bring to a boil. Reduce the heat and simmer for 8 minutes. Remove the chicken from the pot. Cut or pull the meat from the bones. Strain the vegetables from the stock and set aside. Reserve 2 cups of the stock for pot pie; reserve remainder for another use. Combine the olive oil and flour in a large skillet. Whisk over medium heat until the mixture form a roux (a thick paste). Add 2 cups reserved stock gradually and continue to whisk until the sauce has thickened. Add the chicken, vegetables, parsley and tarragon. Pour the chicken mixture into a deep-dish pie pan or casserole. Remove the pastry from the refrigerator and sprinkle both sides with flour. Roll between 2 sheets of waxed paper to form a circle large enough to cover the dish and extend by 1 inch. Remove the waxed paper. Invert the pastry over the filling and crimp the edge. Brush with the reserved 2 tablespoons egg and pierce with a fork several times to vent. Bake for 25 to 30 minutes or until golden brown. ***Serves 4***

Note: Use 1 or 2 tablespoons additional gluten-free flour for a thicker sauce.

Photo for this recipe on page 51.

Gluten-free	Casein-free	Yeast-free

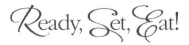
Oven-Roasted Turkey

Preparation Time: 15 minutes   Cooking Time: 1¹/2 hours

2 pounds free-range, antibiotic-free turkey breast
Olive oil
Thyme, organic sea salt and pepper to taste
¹/2 cup chopped celery
¹/2 cup chopped carrots

Preheat the oven to 450 degrees. Drizzle the turkey breast with the olive oil. Brown the turkey breast on both sides in a hot ovenproof skillet. Sprinkle with thyme, salt and pepper. Add the vegetables and drizzle with a small amount of olive oil. Roast for ¹/2 hour per pound for 1 hour. Cover the turkey with aluminum foil for the last 30 minutes of roasting time. Let stand for 10 to 15 minutes for easier slicing. **Serves 8**

Gluten-free	*Casein-free*	*Soy-free*	*Yeast-free*	*Egg-free*

Snappy Gravy: Remove the turkey from the roasting pan. Skim off any fat and strain the turkey stock through a fine sieve onto a bowl. Warm 2 to 3 tablespoons olive oil in a saucepan over medium heat. Add 2 tablespoons Gluten-Free Flour Blend (page 67). Cook for 2 to 3 minutes or until the oil is absorbed, stirring constantly. Gradually add about 2 cups of the reserved turkey stock until creamy, stirring constantly.

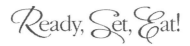

Cod with Spinach and Tomatoes

Preparation Time: 10 minutes   Cooking Time: 15 minutes

1/2 onion, chopped
2 shallots, chopped
3 garlic cloves, chopped
1 tablespoon olive oil
1 (15-ounce) can chopped tomatoes
3 tablespoons tomato paste
1 teaspoon cumin
16 ounces fresh spinach
1 tablespoon olive oil
4 wild cod fillets

Sauté the onion, shallots and garlic in 1 tablespoon olive oil in a medium skillet over medium heat until the onion is golden. Add the tomatoes, tomato paste and cumin and mix well. Simmer for 3 to 5 minutes or until slightly thickened, stirring occasionally. Stir in the spinach. Cook for 2 to 3 minutes. Heat 1 tablespoon olive oil in a large skillet and arrange the cod in the skillet. Cover the cod with the prepared sauce. Simmer for 5 to 8 minutes or until the fish is opaque and flakes easily with a fork. *Serves 4*

Gluten-free	*Casein-free*	*Soy-free*	*Yeast-free*

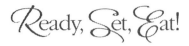

Oven-Roasted Halibut

Preparation Time: 5 minutes   *Cooking Time: 20 minutes*

4   (4-ounce) wild halibut fillets
Organic sea salt and pepper
    to taste
Juice of 1 lemon
5   tablespoons olive oil

3   tablespoons grated Parmesan-flavored
    rice cheese
1   tomato, cut into 1/2-inch pieces
3   garlic cloves, finely chopped
Basil to taste

Preheat the oven to 375 degrees. Place the halibut in a shallow ovenproof dish and sprinkle with salt, pepper and the lemon juice. Top with the olive oil, rice Parmesan cheese, tomato, garlic and basil. Bake for 15 to 18 minutes or until the fish flakes easily. *Serves 4*

Note: You may make **Oven-Roasted Mackeral** by substituting mackeral fillets for the halibut and 1 tablespoon chopped fresh parsley for the rice Parmesan cheese.

Gluten-free   *Casein-free*   *Yeast-free*

Crispy Salmon Nuggets

Preparation Time: 10 minutes   *Cooking Time: 10 minutes*

1   cup gluten-free bread crumbs
2   teaspoons organic sea salt
2   tablespoons dried parsley
1   teaspoon ground cumin (optional)
1/2 cup plain unsweetened almond milk
    or rice milk

2   pounds wild salmon, cut into
    3-inch pieces
1/4 cup extra-virgin olive oil

Mix the bread crumbs, salt, parsley and cumin together in a shallow bowl. Pour the almond milk into a large bowl. Dip the salmon pieces in the milk and then coat in the bread crumb mixture. Heat the olive oil in a shallow skillet. Add the salmon pieces. Fry over medium heat until the center is cooked through or to 160 degrees, turning once. Drain on paper towels. *Serves 8*

Variation: Substitute any hearty, meaty fish such as orange roughy or tilapia for the salmon.

Gluten-free   *Casein-free*   *Yeast-free*

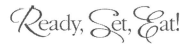

Light Cheese Enchiladas

Preparation Time: 20 minutes   Cooking Time: 3 to 4 minutes

1 yellow onion
8 ounces dairy-free soy-free
mozzarella-flavored cheese substitute*, shredded
4 dried red peppers*
1 garlic clove, minced
Organic sea salt and pepper to taste
Ground cumin to taste*
4 gluten-free corn tortillas
1 tablespoon olive oil
1/2 cup shredded dairy-free soy-free
mozzarella-flavored cheese substitute*

Preheat the oven to 350 degrees. Chop the onion into 1-inch pieces and mix with 8 ounces dairy-free cheese. Soak the peppers in a bowl of cold water for 5 minutes or until soft. Cut lengthwise to remove the seeds. Cut into 2-inch pieces. Heat the peppers and garlic in a small skillet over medium heat for 1 minute. Place in a blender and pulse for 30 seconds to make a paste. Season with salt, pepper and cumin. Spread each tortilla with a thin layer of the pepper paste and heat in a lightly oiled skillet for 30 seconds on each side to soften. Remove the tortillas from the skillet. Fill each with 2 spoonfuls of the onion mixture and roll up to enclose the filling. Place the enchiladas seam side down in a shallow casserole. Sprinkle 1/2 cup mozzarella cheese on top. Bake on the middle oven rack for 1 to 2 minutes or until the cheese is melted. Serve warm. **Serves 4**

Note: You may substitute 1 (16-ounce) can of organic baked pinto or black beans for the cheese filling. Mix the onion with the beans and roll up as above.

Gluten-free   Casein-free   Soy-free   Lactose-free   Cholesterol-free
Good source of protein and calcium

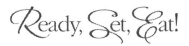

Vegetable Lasagna

Preparation Time: 55 minutes   Cooking Time: 45 minutes

2 eggplant
Organic sea salt
1 pound sliced button mushrooms
1/2 cup extra-virgin olive oil
3 cups gluten-free tomato sauce*
1/2 teaspoon dried basil
1/2 teaspoon dried oregano
9 lasagna noodles*
3 cups shredded dairy-free mozzarella cheese*

Preheat the oven to 375 degrees. Peel the eggplant and cut crosswise into 2-inch slices. Salt generously on both sides and place in a large colander. Let stand for 15 minutes or until small drops of water appear on the surface of the eggplant. Rinse and pat dry with a paper towel. Place the eggplant and mushrooms on a large baking sheet brushed with some of the olive oil. Brush the top of vegetables with olive oil. Roast for about 30 minutes, flipping the vegetables halfway through the cooking process. Mix the tomato sauce with the basil and oregano in a bowl. Spread 3/4 cup of the tomato sauce in a 9×13-inch baking dish. Place 3 lasagna noodles crosswise over the sauce, leaving about 1 inch between them as they expand during cooking. Spread 1 cup of the cheese over the pasta. Spread another 3/4 cup of the tomato sauce over the cheese followed by a layer of eggplant and mushrooms. Repeat the layers until all the ingredients are used, ending with a layer of cheese. Bake, covered with foil, for 30 minutes. Remove the foil and bake for 10 to 15 minutes longer or until the cheese is golden. Let stand for 5 minutes before serving. *Serves 8 to 10*

Note: You can store extra pasta pieces, wrapped in plastic wrap, in a cool dry place for future use.

Gluten-free   Casein-free   Yeast-free

Manicotti

Preparation Time: 30 minutes   Cooking Time: 30 minutes

Crepes

2 free-range eggs, beaten
1 cup milk alternative, such as plain rice milk
1/2 teaspoon organic sea salt
1 cup all-purpose Gluten-Free Flour Blend (page 67)
Olive oil

Combine the eggs, milk alternative, salt and Flour Blend in a bowl and stir until smooth. Cover and let stand for 30 minutes. Heat a 5- or 6-inch frying pan that has been lightly greased with olive oil. Pour in 2 tablespoons of the batter and tilt and swirl to coat the bottom of the pan. Cook on one side for 1 minute. Flip with a spatula and cook the other side. Plate the crepe and repeat with the remaining batter.

Filling

2 cups shredded dairy-free, soy-free cheese*
1 free-range egg
Organic sea salt and pepper to taste
Crepes
1 cup gluten-free spaghetti sauce

Preheat the oven to 375 degrees. Mix the cheese, egg, salt and pepper in a bowl. Place 1 tablespoon of the filling on each crepe and gently roll up. Spread enough spaghetti sauce to cover the bottom of a 9×12-inch baking pan. Arrange the filled crepes over the sauce and pour more sauce over the top. Bake, covered, for 30 minutes. *Serves 15 to 18*

Note: The recommended cheese contains inactive yeast. Please call the company to receive further information.

Gluten-free   Casein-free   Soy-free

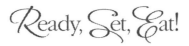

Hearty Vegetarian Tacos

Preparation Time: 15 minutes

1 large Haas avocado
1 tablespoon lemon juice
1 garlic clove, chopped
1/2 cup chopped fresh tomato
1 tablespoon gluten-free salsa seasoning*
3 tablespoons chopped fresh cilantro
1 (16-ounce) can organic green wasabi peas, drained
1 cup chopped fresh romaine
1/2 cup shredded Cheddar-flavored dairy-free cheese*
1 cup soy sour cream*
6 to 8 corn taco shells

Mash the avocado in a mixing bowl with a fork. Mix in the lemon juice, garlic, tomato, salsa seasoning and cilantro. Set the table with bowls of the wasabi peas, lettuce, cheese and sour cream. Build your own tacos by filling the taco shells with your favorite toppings.
Serves 4 or 5

Tip: This is a light and delicious lunch that is easy to prepare with no cooking involved so you can spend more time with your family.

Gluten-free	Casein-free	Yeast-free	Egg-free

Genetically Modified Organisms: Since no one outside the GMO industry has conducted independent research proving the safety of GMOs for human consumption, we are unable to predict their long-term effects on health. What we do know is that GMO plants do not have the genetic makeup of their naturally occurring counterpart. Therefore, it stands to reason that the GMO plant will not behave in the body in the same way as its natural counterpart. Since about 70% of all corn produced is GMO based, the only GMO-free corn chip or Taco would be a certified organic kind.

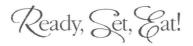

Pasta Primavera with Vegetables

Preparation Time: 5 minutes   Cooking Time: 15 minutes

8 cups water
2 teaspoons organic sea salt
8 ounces gluten-free corkscrew pasta (rotini)
1/2 cup chopped roasted red pepper
1/2 cup chopped artichoke hearts
1 teaspoon organic sea salt
2 to 3 tablespoons cold-pressed extra-virgin olive oil
2 basil leaves (optional)

Bring the water and 2 teaspoons salt to a boil in a large pot. Add the pasta and cook for about 8 minutes. Drain and rinse the pasta. Add the vegetables to the cooked pasta. Add 1 teaspoon salt and the olive oil and toss to mix. Roll the basil leaves into a cigar shape and chop crosswise into a chiffonade. Sprinkle over the pasta. *Serves 8*

Gluten-free	*Casein-free*	*Yeast-free*

Baked Ziti

Preparation Time: 10 minutes   Cooking Time: 40 minutes

1 pound quinoa rotelle
1 pinch of organic sea salt
1 pound gluten-free bulk Italian sausage
16 ounces gluten-free pasta sauce
1 pinch of gluten-free red pepper flakes
1/2 teaspoon ground black pepper
2 teaspoons dried basil
16 ounces shredded mozzarella-flavored dairy-free cheese*

Preheat the oven to 400 degrees. Bring a large pot of water to boil. Add the pasta and salt. Cook the pasta for about 10 minutes or until al dente; drain and set aside. Crumble the sausage using your fingers and brown in a small skillet over medium heat. Mix together the sausage, pasta sauce, red pepper flakes, ground pepper, dried basil and half the cheese in a bowl. Spoon the pasta into a 9×13-inch baking dish and cover with the sausage mixture. Sprinkle with the remaining cheese. Bake for about 30 minutes or until lightly golden on top. Serve warm. *Serves 6*

Note: You may use fresh mozzarella cheese if not casein intolerant.

Photo for this recipe on page 54.

Gluten-free	*Casein-free*	*Yeast-free*	*Soy-free*	*Egg-free*

Cookies and Desserts

The Recipes

Easy and Elegant Brownies

Preparation Time: 10 minutes   *Baking Time: 30 minutes*

1   cup butter substitute
4   ounces unsweetened chocolate
1   cup organic dark brown sugar
1¹/2 cups Gluten-Free Flour Blend
    (page 67)
4   free-range eggs (see note below)

1   teaspoon organic sea salt
1   teaspoon baking powder
2   teaspoons gluten-free vanilla extract*
1   cup semisweet gluten-free, dairy-free
    chocolate chips*

Preheat the oven to 350 degrees. Melt the butter substitute and unsweetened chocolate in a medium saucepan over medium heat, stirring frequently. Stir in the brown sugar, Flour Blend, eggs, salt, baking powder and vanilla. Fold in the chocolate chips and pour into a greased 9×13-inch baking pan. Bake on the middle oven rack for about 30 to 32 minutes. *Serves 8*

Note: Organic dark brown sugar is soft, moist sugar that has not been filtered through animal by-products and is suitable for Vegan, Vegetarian, Halal, and Plant-based diets. This dark sugar is perfect for brownies, gingerbread, or rich chocolate-based desserts.

Photo for this recipe on page 49.

Gluten-free	*Casein-free*	*Egg-free (see note)*	*Nut-free*

Chocolate Chip Cookies

Preparation Time: 15 minutes   *Baking Time: 13 minutes*

1¹/2 cups Gluten-Free Flour Blend
    (page 67)
1/4 teaspoon xanthan gum
1/2 teaspoon baking soda
1/2 teaspoon organic sea salt
1/2 cup dairy-free butter substitute*
1/2 cup packed organic dark brown sugar

2   free-range eggs (see note below)
1/2 teaspoon gluten-free vanilla extract
3/4 cup gluten-free, casein-free
    chocolate chips*
1   cup chopped walnuts or pecans
    (optional)

Preheat the oven to 350 degrees. Combine the Flour Blend, xanthan gum, baking soda and salt in a large bowl and mix well. Cream the butter substitute and brown sugar in a small bowl. Mix in the eggs and vanilla. Stir the egg mixture into the flour mixture gradually. Stir in the chocolate chips and walnuts. Drop by teaspoonfuls onto a greased cookie sheet. Bake for 10 to 13 minutes. Remove from the cookie sheet while still hot and place on wire racks to cool. *Makes 12*

Gluten-free	*Casein-free*	*Yeast-free*	*Egg-free (see note)*

Note: If you are egg allergic, use egg substitute.

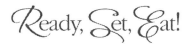

Chocolate Chippers

Preparation Time: 15 minutes   *Baking Time: 10 to 12 minutes*

1   cup rice flour
$^1/_3$ cup gluten-free, dairy-free
    chocolate chips*
$1^1/_2$ teaspoons egg replacer, or
    1 free-range egg*

2   tablespoons water
2   tablespoons canola oil
$^1/_4$ cup pure maple syrup
1   teaspoon gluten-free vanilla*
2   teaspoons canola oil

Preheat the oven to 350 degrees. Place the rice flour in a bowl and mix in the chocolate chips. Mix the egg replacer with 2 tablespoons water in a small bowl. Add 2 tablespoons canola oil, the maple syrup and vanilla; add to the rice flour. Mix well and shape into a ball. Chill for 1 hour or longer. Oil a large cookie sheet with 2 teaspoons canola oil. Shape the cookie dough into 1-inch balls and place on the prepared cookie sheet. Press with the bottom of a glass or cup to flatten. Bake for 10 to 12 minutes or until golden. *Makes 12 to 14*

Gluten-free	Casein-free	Yeast-free	Egg-free	Nut-free

Coconut Almond Sugar Cookies

Preparation Time: 20 minutes   *Baking Time: 10 to 12 minutes per batch*

1   cup beet sugar
$^1/_2$ cup softened coconut oil
$^1/_3$ cup plain rice milk
2   teaspoons gluten-free vanilla extract
$^3/_4$ cup white rice flour
$^1/_3$ cup coconut flour

2   tablespoons potato starch,
    tapioca starch, or tapioca flour
$^1/_2$ teaspoon baking powder
$^1/_2$ teaspoon baking soda
$^1/_2$ cup ground organic almonds

Preheat the oven to 350 degrees. Pour the sugar into a mixing bowl. Add the coconut oil 1 tablespoon at a time and beat for 1 minute or until blended after each addition. Add the rice milk and vanilla and beat for 1 minute. Combine the rice flour, coconut flour, potato starch, baking powder and baking soda in a bowl and mix well. Add the dry ingredients to the coconut oil mixture and beat for 1 minute. Add the almonds and beat lightly for 10 seconds. The mixture should be moist and fluffy. Drop by rounded tablespoonfuls on a greased cookie sheet. Bake for 10 to 12 minutes or until golden. *Makes 24*

Note: Coconut oil gives added coconut flavor to these delicious cookies in addition to its beneficial medium-chain fatty acids. Interestingly, these cookies contain no cholesterol and only about 10 grams of sugar per cookie, so you can enjoy them guilt-free! You may keep these cookies up to 1 week in an airtight container.

Gluten-free	Casein-free	Yeast-free	Soy-free

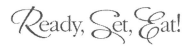

Scrumptious Cranberry Cookies

Preparation Time: 30 minutes   *Baking Time: 20 minutes*

1/2 cup butter substitute*, softened
1/2 cup packed light brown sugar
1/2 cup beet sugar
2   free-range eggs
1   teaspoon almond extract
2   cups gluten-free all-purpose flour

1   teaspoon organic sea salt
1/4 teaspoon baking powder
1   cup sliced almonds, toasted
1/2 cup unsweetened sun-dried
     organic cranberries

Preheat the oven to 300 degrees. Cream the butter substitute with the brown sugar and beet sugar in a bowl with an electric mixer until fluffy. Add the eggs and almond extract and beat at low speed until well combined. Sift the flour, salt and baking powder into a bowl. Beat into the butter mixture at low speed, stopping the mixer once to scrape down the sides. Stir in the almonds and cranberries. Drop by large tablespoonfuls 2 inches apart onto a greased cookie sheet and flatten slightly. Bake for 20 minutes or until golden. Cool on wire racks. ***Makes 24***

Photo for this recipe on page 52.

Gluten-free	Casein-free	Yeast-free

Crunchy Granola Bars

Preparation Time: 10 minutes   *Baking Time: 40 to 45 minutes*

1   cup sliced raw organic almonds
2   cups gluten-free oats
1/2 cup pure maple syrup
2/3 cup local raw honey
11/2 teaspoons gluten-free vanilla extract

1   teaspoon organic sea salt
1/2 cup chopped dried organic
     cranberries
3   tablespoons coconut oil
     (or dairy-free butter substitute*)

Preheat the oven to 325 degrees. Line a large rimmed baking pan with baking parchment. Toast the almonds and oats together in a large nonstick skillet over medium heat for 3 to 4 minutes or until the mixture is slightly brown. Mix the maple syrup, honey, vanilla, salt, cranberries and coconut oil in a bowl. Add the oats mixture and mix well. Pour into the prepared baking pan and press with the back of a spoon. Bake on the middle oven rack for 40 to 45 minutes or until golden brown. Cook for about 1 hour before cutting into individual bars. ***Makes 12***

Gluten-free	Casein-free	Egg-free	Soy-free	Yeast-free

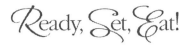

Peanut Butter Cookies

Preparation Time: 5 minutes   Baking Time: 12 minutes

2 free-range eggs, or equivalent amount of egg substitute
1 cup chunky peanut butter or almond butter
1 cup beet sugar

Preheat the oven to 350 degrees. Beat the eggs in a bowl. Stir in the peanut butter and sugar until well mixed. Drop by teaspoonfuls onto a greased cookie sheet and flatten with a fork. Bake for 10 to 12 minutes. ***Makes 24***

Gluten-free	*Casein-free*	*Yeast-free*	*Lactose-free*	*Soy-free*

Beet sugar is derived from sugar beets and is 99.9 percent pure sucrose. Each teaspoon contains only 15 calories and 4 grams of beet sugar (20 percent fewer grams than table sugar). Sucrose turns into energy, causing no insulin surge in moderation (great for diabetics). It's a good substitute for other sweeteners such as barley malt, date sugar, fructose, dextrose, and xylitol.

Austrian Linzer Cookies

Preparation Time: 20 minutes   Baking Time: 20 minutes

3¹/₂ tablespoons butter substitute*,
    softened
2¹/₂ tablespoons beet sugar
¹/₈ teaspoon organic sea salt
¹/₄ cup finely ground hazelnuts
2   tablespoons finely ground almonds
1   free-range egg yolk

¹/₈ teaspoon gluten-free vanilla extract
¹/₃ cup plus 1 tablespoon Gluten-Free
    Flour Blend (page 67), sifted
Rice flour
6   tablespoons seedless raspberry jam
¹/₃ cup organic confectioners'
    sugar, sifted

Preheat the oven to 375 degrees. Combine the butter, sugar, salt, hazelnuts, almonds, egg yolk and vanilla in a mixing bowl and beat until smooth. Add the Flour Blend and mix well. Shape the dough into a ball and wrap in plastic wrap. Chill for about 1 hour. Roll out the dough to about ¹/₆-inch thickness on a surface dusted with rice flour. Use a round 2-inch cookie cutter to cut out 20 circles of dough for the cookie bottoms. Cut out 20 more with fluted 2-inch cutter for the cookie tops. Cut a 1-inch hole in the center of each fluted circle. Place the dough circles on a greased cookie sheet and bake for 20 minutes or until golden; cool completely. Drop a quarter-size amount of jam onto each cookie bottom. Place the cookie tops on waxed paper and dust with the confectioners' sugar. Place the tops on the jam-filled cookie bottoms. ***Makes 20***

Note: These are one of Austria's most famous desserts. The nutty flavor and sweet jam makes them extra special. Best of all, two cookies render only four grams of sugar!

Gluten-free	*Yeast-free*

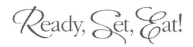

French Madeleines

Preparation Time: 15 minutes   *Baking Time: 8 to 12 minutes*

Melted butter substitute* for coating
5   free-range eggs
1/2 cup beet sugar
1/2 cup butter substitute*, melted
1   teaspoon gluten-free vanilla extract

Zest of 1 lemon or orange
11/2 cups gluten-free all-purpose flour*
1/4 teaspoon xanthan gum
1   teaspoon baking powder
Confectioners' sugar

Preheat the oven to 400 degrees. Coat the madeleine pans generously with melted butter. Beat the eggs in a bowl until light yellow in color. Add the sugar, 1/2 cup butter, the vanilla and lemon zest and mix well. Mix the flour, xanthan gum and baking powder together in a bowl. Add the egg mixture and mix well; do not overmix. Place about 1 tablespoon batter into each madeleine mold. Bake for 8 to 12 minutes or until light golden in color. Turn out and cool. Dust with confectioners' sugar. *Makes 12*

Gluten-free   *Yeast-free*

Delicious Peanut Butter
Oatmeal Cranberry Cookies

Preparation Time: 20 minutes   *Baking Time: 12 to 15 minutes*

Gluten-free rolled oats
1/2 cup raw honey
1/3 cup packed brown sugar
1/2 cup coconut oil, softened
1/2 cup peanut butter
1/2 teaspoon gluten-free vanilla extract

1   cup rice flour
1   teaspoon baking soda
1/4 teaspoon organic sea salt (optional)
1/2 cup organic dried cranberries
    (optional)

Preheat the oven to 350 degrees. Process enough gluten-free rolled oats in a food processor or blender to yield 3/4 cup oat flour. Combine the honey, brown sugar, coconut oil, peanut butter and vanilla in a medium bowl until creamy. Combine the oat flour, rice flour, baking soda and salt in a small bowl. Add to the peanut butter mixture and mix well. Stir in the craisins. Drop by rounded teaspoonfuls about 2 inches apart onto an ungreased cookie sheet. Bake for 12 to 15 minutes or until light golden brown. Cool for 3 to 5 minutes before removing from the cookie sheet. *Makes 36*

Note: Store any leftovers in an airtight container in the freezer for up to one week.

Gluten-free   *Casein-free*   *Yeast-free*   *Soy-free*

Pecan Cookies

Preparation Time: 30 minutes   *Baking Time: 10 to 12 minutes*

3/4 cup packed brown sugar
1/2 cup margarine or butter substitute*, softened
2 medium free-range eggs, beaten

1 cup potato starch*
1/2 cup pure rice flour*
1/2 cup crushed pecans

Preheat oven to 375 degrees. Cream the brown sugar and margarine in a bowl. Mix in the eggs until smooth. Add the potato starch and rice flour and mix well. Mix in the pecans. Drop by tablespoonfuls onto a greased cookie sheet. Bake for 10 to 12 minutes or until golden brown. *Makes 2 dozen*

Gluten-free

Crispy Rice Balls

Preparation Time: 30 minutes

1/2 cup gluten-free marshmallow creme*
4 cups crisp rice cereal*
1 teaspoon light cooking oil

Combine the marshmallow creme and cereal in a large bowl and mix with a plastic spatula. Grease your hands with the oil. Shape small amounts of the cereal mixture into balls. *Makes about 1 dozen*

Variation: Roll the rice balls in chopped roasted pecans or walnuts if not allergic to tree nuts.

Gluten-free	*Casein-free*	*Yeast-free*	*Soy-free*	*Egg-free*

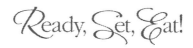

Almond Banana Split

Preparation Time: 15 minutes

2 large organic bananas (no brown spots)
2 tablespoons creamy organic almond butter
10 miniature chocolate chips*

Peel and split the bananas lengthwise. Place cut sides down on serving plates. Spread 1 tablespoon of the almond butter on the outer side of two of the banana halves. Attach 2 half bananas so the sticky sides are connected. Place the attached banana halves in 2 large ice cream bowls. Sprinkle the top of each banana split with 5 miniature chocolate chips. **Serves 2**

Note: This is a great afternoon snack for children or adults who don't like plain fruit. By adding the almond butter, you are adding beneficial vegetable protein, healthy fat, and several necessary minerals such as iron, magnesium, manganese, and vitamins B1 and biotin while providing less than 5 grams of sugar per serving. A touch of chocolate, preferably dark, is a great source of antioxidants (8 times higher than strawberries) and flavonoids, which are thought to lower blood pressure and balance certain hormones. Remember, damage control through portion control!

Gluten-free	*Casein-free*	*Yeast-free*	*Egg-free*	*Soy-free*

Apple Pecan Crisp

Preparation Time: 30 minutes *Baking Time: 15 to 20 minutes*

2 pounds golden Delicious apples, peeled and chopped into 1-inch pieces
1/2 teaspoon organic sea salt
1/2 teaspoon cinnamon
1/4 cup packed organic light brown sugar
1 tablespoon butter substitute*, melted

1 tablespoon arrowroot
1/4 cup water
1/2 cup almond flour
1/4 cup packed organic light brown sugar
1 tablespoon butter substitute*, softened
1/2 cup chopped pecans
Dairy-free vanilla ice cream

Preheat the oven to 375 degrees. Mix the apples, salt, cinnamon, 1/4 cup brown sugar and melted butter in a bowl. Blend the arrowroot and water in a small bowl. Toss with the apples. Spoon into a baking dish. Mix the almond flour, 1/4 cup brown sugar and softened butter in a small bowl until crumbly. Sprinkle over the apple mixture. Top with the pecans. Bake for 15 minutes or until golden on top and bubbly around the edges. Cool on a wire rack. Serve with ice cream, if desired. **Serves 6**

Variation: You may substitute organic blueberries and peaches for the apples, if desired.

Gluten-free	*Dairy-free*	*Egg-free*

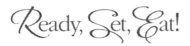

Berry Crumble

Preparation Time: 30 minutes   *Baking Time: 30 to 35 minutes*

2   cups frozen organic blueberries
1   cup frozen organic blackberries
1   tablespoon blue agave nectar*
2   tablespoons fresh-squeezed lime juice
1   cup blanched almond flour*

$^1/_2$ cup gluten-free oats*
$^1/_2$ teaspoon cinnamon
$^1/_2$ teaspoon nutmeg
$^1/_2$ cup butter substitute*, softened
$^1/_2$ cup blue agave nectar*

Preheat the oven to 375 degrees. Grease a 9×13-inch baking pan with coconut oil. Combine the blueberries, blackberries, 1 tablespoon agave nectar and the lime juice in a bowl and toss until the fruit is coated. Spoon into the prepared baking pan. Combine the almond flour, oats, cinnamon and nutmeg in a bowl. Combine the butter and $^1/_2$ cup agave nectar in a bowl and mix well. Cut into the flour mixture until crumbly. Sprinkle over the berries. Bake for 30 to 35 minutes or until cooked through and bubbly. Serve as dessert or breakfast. **Serves 6**

Photo for this recipe on page 52.

Gluten-free	Casein-free	Egg-free

Bûche de Noël

Preparation Time: 20 minutes   *Baking Time: 20 minutes*

4   free-range eggs, separated
$^1/_4$ cup coconut oil
$^1/_2$ cup water
2   cups gluten-free chocolate cake mix

1   (4-ounce) package firm tofu
$^1/_4$ cup water
1   (4-ounce) package vegan vanilla
    cream pudding mix*

Preheat the oven to 350 degrees. Whip the egg whites in a bowl to soft peaks. Beat the egg yolks in a bowl. Fold into the egg whites. Mix in the next 3 ingredients. Do not beat; the batter should remain fluffy. Spoon into a waxed paper-lined 10×15-inch baking pan. Bake for 18 minutes or until the cake bounces back when lightly touched. Let stand until slightly cooled. Place the cake with the waxed-paper side down on a clean damp kitchen towel. Roll as for a jelly roll; cool on a wire rack. Process the tofu and $^1/_4$ cup water in a food processor until smooth. Add the pudding mix and process until creamy. Unroll the cooled cake; remove the towel and waxed paper. Spread the vanilla filling to within 2 inches of the short edges and then reroll. Place seam side down on a serving plate. You may also cut the cake vertically into 3 equal strips. Alternate layers of cake and vanilla filling, ending with the filling. Chill for 15 minutes before serving. Garnish as desired with berries, mint leaves or holly leaves made with almond paste. **Serves 6 to 8**

Photo for this recipe on page 51.

Gluten-free	Yeast-free

Angel Food Cake

Preparation Time: 15 minutes   *Baking Time: 35 to 40 minutes*

Gluten-Free Flour Mix:

2 cups gluten-free white rice flour
2/3 cup gluten-free potato starch flour
1/3 cup gluten-free tapioca flour

Combine the rice flour, potato starch flour and tapioca flour in a bowl and mix well. Store in an airtight container.

Cake:

1 cup plus 2 tablespoons Gluten-Free Flour Mix (above)
1/2 cup beet sugar
1/4 teaspoon organic sea salt
1/4 teaspoon xanthan gum
12 free-range egg whites
1 1/2 teaspoons cream of tartar
1 1/2 teaspoons gluten-free vanilla extract
3/4 cup beet sugar

Preheat the oven to 350 degrees. Combine the Flour Mix, 1/2 cup sugar, the salt and xanthan gum in a bowl until smooth. Blend the egg whites with the cream of tartar and vanilla in a mixing bowl. Add 3/4 cup sugar gradually, beating until stiff peaks form. Fold the flour mixture into the egg mixture until blended. Pour the batter into an ungreased 10-inch tube pan. Bake for 35 to 40 minutes or until golden brown. Invert onto a wire rack and let cool until the cake feels spongy. Loosen the cake from the side of the pan and invert onto a serving plate. *Serves 8*

Note: Top this delicious but light cake with sliced fresh organic strawberries for a beautiful presentation.

Gluten-free	*Casein-free*	*Soy-free*	*Yeast-free*

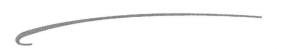

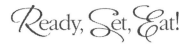

Perfect Vanilla Cupcakes

Preparation Time: 20 minutes   *Baking Time: 25 minutes*

1   cup beet sugar
3   large free-range eggs
2   teaspoons gluten-free vanilla extract
2/3 cup coconut oil
3¼ cups gluten-free flour
1   tablespoon baking powder
1   teaspoon baking soda

1   teaspoon xanthan gum
1   teaspoon organic sea salt
1   teaspoon gluten-free cider vinegar or
    lemon juice
1¹/₃ cups rice milk
Sliced almonds

Preheat the oven to 350 degrees. Combine the sugar, eggs, vanilla and coconut oil in a large bowl. Beat for 2 minutes or until thick. Mix the flour, baking powder, baking soda, xanthan gum and salt in a bowl. Combine the vinegar and rice milk in a small bowl. Fold the flour mixture and rice milk mixture alternately into the egg mixture one-half at a time, mixing well after each addition. Spoon into paper-lined muffin cups. Sprinkle with sliced almonds. Bake for 20 to 25 minutes or until golden brown. ***Makes 22 cupcakes***

Note: These cupcakes are perfect for birthdays or any special occasion.

Photo for this recipe on page 52.

Gluten-free	*Soy-free*	*Yeast-free*	*Casein-free*

Frosting

Preparation Time: 10 minutes

1 free-range egg white
1 cup confectioners' sugar
3 tablespoons rice milk or
unsweetened vanilla-flavored almond milk

Beat the egg white in a mixing bowl until frothy. Add the confectioners' sugar and milk and beat until the frosting is thick and spreadable. ***Makes about 1¹/₂ cups***

Variation: For egg-free frosting, combine 1 cup softened coconut oil, 1 cup confectioners' sugar and 1 teaspoon gluten-free vanilla extract in a bowl. Beat for 1 minute on medium speed; use immediately.

Editor's Note: If you are concerned about using raw egg whites, use whites from eggs pasteurized in their shells, or use the equivalent amount of powdered egg whites and follow the package directions.

Gluten-free	*Casein-free*	*Soy-free*	*Yeast-free*

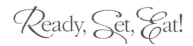

Delightful Ice Cream

Preparation Time: 30 minutes   Freezing Time: up to 3 hours

6 cups unsweetened original almond milk
2 teaspoons gluten-free vanilla extract
1 cup chopped pitted Madjdool dates
1/2 cup unfiltered raw honey*
1/4 cup cold-pressed coconut oil

Combine all the ingredients in an electric blender and process until smooth. Pour into a glass freezer-safe bowl. Freeze, uncovered, for 1 hour. Stir to ensure a smooth final product and return to the freezer. **Makes 1 quart**

Option: Pour the mixture into an ice cream maker and follow the manufacturer's instructions.

Gluten-free	Casein-free	Soy-free	Yeast-free	Egg-free

Silky Coconut Ice Cream

Preparation Time: 30 minutes   Freezing Time: up to 5 hours

6 cups vanilla-flavored coconut milk
1 cup chopped pitted Madjdool dates
1/2 cup unfiltered raw honey*
1/4 cup cold-pressed coconut oil

Combine all the ingredients in an electric blender and process until smooth. Pour into an ice cream maker and following the manufacturer's instructions. **Makes 1 quart**

Variation: For those not allergic to tree nuts, replace the coconut milk with unsweetened almond milk and add 2 teaspoons gluten-free vanilla extract. Mix as directed above.

Photo for this recipe on page 55.

Gluten-free	Casein-free	Soy-free	Yeast-free	Egg-free

Virgin Coconut Oil Is King! This richly flavored tropical oil is very useful in baking as a substitute for butter as it produces very moist baked goods such as cakes and cupcakes. Compared to other vegetable oils, coconut oil has a high smoke point, making it a great for light cooking and frying as well.

Coconut Ice Cream Sandwiches

Preparation Time: 5 minutes

8 Chocolate Chippers (page 118)
1 pint gluten-free coconut ice cream*

Place the cookies flat side up on a cookie sheet or flat tray. Place a scoop of ice cream on one cookie and spread evenly to about 2 inches thick. Place another cookie flat side down over the ice cream layer. Repeat with the remaining ingredients. Serve immediately. *Serves 4*

Variation: Toast 1/2 cup chopped hazelnuts in a nonstick pan over medium heat for 1 minute. Roll the ice cream sandwiches sideways in a plate of toasted hazelnuts to coat the ice cream. This will help add good unsaturated fats to your diet.

Note: This is a quick dessert recipe that puts a smile on everyone's face. Whether you want to lose weight or watch your waist line, control the sugar intake by making smaller cookies and spreading a thinner layer of ice cream.

Gluten-free	*Casein-free*	*Soy-free*	*Yeast-free*

Berry Sorbet

Preparation Time: 90 minutes

2	cups fresh organic raspberries	1	cup organic orange sections
1	cup fresh organic strawberries, hulled	2	organic peaches, peeled and sliced
1/4	cup fresh orange juice	1	teaspoon gluten-free vanilla extract

Combine the raspberries, strawberries, orange juice, orange sections, peaches and vanilla in a blender. Process until smooth. Transfer the puréed fruit to an ice cream maker. Prepare according to the manufacturer's instructions or spoon into an ice tray and freeze for at least 1 hour. Stir every 30 minutes or purée in a blender before serving. Spoon into individual serving dishes and garnish with a mint leaf and additional raspberries. *Serves 6*

Note: This is a refreshing sorbet rich in antioxidants. You may use frozen organic berries and bottled organic peaches if fresh are unavailable.

Gluten-free	*Casein-free*	*Egg-free*	*Yeast-free*	*Nut-free*

Custard Peach Pie

Preparation Time: 10 minutes   Baking Time: 20 minutes

2 cups sliced peeled organic peaches
2 tablespoons beet sugar*
1 tablespoon arrowroot powder*
1/8 teaspoon ground nutmeg
2 tablespoons beet sugar*
1/2 cup soy sour cream*
1 teaspoon gluten-free vanilla extract*
1 free-range egg
1 (9-inch) Crunchy Coconut Pie Crust (page 130)

Preheat the oven to 375 degrees. Combine the peaches, 2 tablespoons sugar, the arrowroot powder and nutmeg in a bowl and toss lightly to coat. Combine 2 tablespoons sugar, the sour cream, vanilla and egg in a small bowl and blend well. Spoon the sour cream mixture into the Pie Crust. Arrange the peaches over the top in a fan shape. Bake for 20 minutes. Garnish with mint sprigs. *Serves 6 to 8*

Tip: The combination of multiple textures and colors of the coconut and almond crust with soft peaches makes this a refreshing summer pie to show off to friends and family for years to come.

Photo for this recipe on page 55.

Gluten-free	*Casein-free*	*Yeast-free*	*Lactose-free*

Note: Peaches, number 1 on the Dirty Dozen list in 2009, ranked number 2 in 2010, with 62 pesticide residues found on peaches. Use organic peaches if possible to avoid pesticide toxicity.

Pumpkin Chiffon Pie

Preparation Time: 15 minutes   Baking Time: 20 minutes

3 free-range egg yolks
1/2 cup beet sugar
1 1/4 cups canned organic pumpkin
1/2 cup coconut milk
1/2 teaspoon organic sea salt
1/2 teaspoon ginger
1/2 teaspoon cinnamon
1/2 teaspoon nutmeg
1 tablespoon or 1 envelope unflavored gelatin
1/4 cup cold water
3 free-range egg whites
1/2 cup beet sugar
1 (9-inch) Crunchy Coconut Pie Crust (page 130)
Whipped cream

Beat the egg yolks and 1/2 cup sugar in a mixing bowl until thick and lemon-colored.
Add the pumpkin, coconut milk, salt and spices to the egg mixture and blend well.
Pour into a double boiler. Cook over simmering water until thickened, stirring constantly.
Soften the gelatin in the cold water. Stir into the hot mixture. Beat the egg whites in a
mixing bowl. Add 1/2 cup sugar gradually, beating until stiff peaks form. Fold into the
pumpkin mixture. Pour into the Pie Crust. Chill until serving time. Top with whipped cream
to serve. ***Serves 6 to 8***

Tip: This easy and elegant dessert is perfect at Thanksgiving or Christmas.

Photo for this recipe on page 50.

Gluten-free	*Casein-free*	*Lactose-free*	*Yeast-free*

Coconut Milk and Yogurt: Coconut milk and other coconut by-products are great
substitutes for dairy in recipes as coconut is sweet, yet low in sugar and rich in good
medium-chain fatty acids. I recommend 1 to 2 cups per day of the unsweetened version
to fit my daily rule of 30 grams of sugar for children and 40 grams for adults. My favorite
brand is also dairy-free, lactose-free, soy-free, gluten-free, a source of vitamin B12, high in
calcium absorption, cholesterol-free, trans fat-free, and certified vegan.

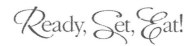

Fresh Strawberry Pie

Preparation Time: 10 minutes   *Chilling Time: 30 minutes or longer*

3/4 cup organic strawberries, hulled
1/2 cup beet sugar
2 tablespoons arrowroot powder
1/2 cup water
1/4 teaspoon organic sea salt

1/2 teaspoon almond extract*
1 (9-inch) Crunchy Coconut Pie Crust (below)
2 1/4 cups organic strawberries, hulled

Mash 3/4 cup strawberries with a fork in a bowl. Mix the sugar and arrowroot powder in a 2-quart saucepan. Stir in the mashed strawberries and water. Cook over medium heat for about 5 minutes, stirring frequently. The mixture will thicken as it comes to a boil. Stir in the salt and almond extract and set aside to cool. Fill the Pie Crust with 2 1/4 cups strawberries and pour the cooked strawberries around them. Refrigerate for 30 minutes or until set. *Serves 8*

Note: Enjoy this refreshing strawberry pie with a dollop of coconut yogurt on top. For a quick dessert, prepare the pie crust ahead of time and freeze. Thaw for about one hour before filling, and it will be ready to serve as soon as the strawberry filling sets.

Photo for this recipe on page 55.

Gluten-free	Casein-free	Egg-free	Yeast-free	Lactose-free

Crunchy Coconut Pie Crust

Preparation Time: 10 minutes   *Cooking Time: 10 minutes*

3/4 cup shredded unsweetened organic coconut
1 cup chopped slivered organic almonds
1/3 teaspoon organic sea salt

1/3 cup plus 1 tablespoon organic coconut oil*
1 tablespoon blue agave nectar*
1 teaspoon gluten-free vanilla extract*

Preheat the oven to 350 degrees. Spread the coconut in a thin layer on an ungreased baking sheet and toast on the middle rack of the oven for 1 minute or until golden. Watch carefully, as coconut can burn easily. Mix the almonds, toasted coconut and salt in a bowl. Blend the coconut oil, nectar and vanilla in a small bowl. Stir into the toasted coconut mixture, mixing well. Press the dough into two (4-inch) pie pans or one (9-inch) tart pan with a removable bottom. Bake for about 10 minutes. Cool before filling. *Makes 1 (9-inch) crust, or 2 (4-inch) crusts*

Note: Chopped almonds and toasted coconut create a delightful crust for a refreshing summer pie.

Gluten-free	Casein-free	Egg-free	Yeast-free	Lactose-free

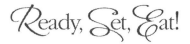

Lemon Pudding with Granola Topping

Preparation Time: 10 minutes

1 (4-ounce) package silken light tofu (firm)
¼ cup water
1 (4-ounce) package vegan lemon cream pudding mix
Crunchy Granola Bar (page 119), chopped

Blend the tofu and water in a blender until creamy. Add the pudding mix and blend until smooth. Pour into individual serving dishes. Sprinkle with Crunchy Granola. *Serves 4*

| *Casein-free* | *Egg-free* | *Lactose-free* | *Yeast-free* |

Rice Pudding

Preparation Time: 5 minutes   *Cooking Time: 20 minutes*

¼ cup white rice starch
2 cups organic coconut milk*
2 tablespoons rose water
¼ cup beet sugar

Combine the rice starch, coconut milk, rose water and sugar in a saucepan. Cook over medium heat for 20 minutes or until of a creamy consistency, stirring frequently with a wooden spoon. Remove from the heat and spoon into a serving bowl. Chill in the refrigerator. *Serves 4*

Note: This silky, light recipe has a floral flavor that reminds me of the scent of fresh blooming spring flowers. Enjoy after a light dinner or as a snack by itself. This recipe is a great source of medium-chain fatty acids and has an anti-fungal effect from the coconut milk. If strictly watching your sugar intake, use Stevia instead of beet sugar.

| *Gluten-free* | *Casein-free* | *Soy-free* | *Yeast-free* |

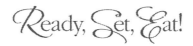

Tapioca Coconut Pudding

Preparation Time: 10 minutes   *Cooking Time: 15 to 20 minutes*

¹/₂ cup tapioca pearls
5 cups coconut milk
6 drops of liquid Stevia (or as needed)
¹/₂ teaspoon gluten-free vanilla extract
³/₄ teaspoon organic sea salt

Place the tapioca, coconut milk and salt in a 2-quart saucepan. Bring to a boil, stirring constantly. Reduce the heat to low and simmer for about 20 minutes, stirring frequently. Add the Stevia and vanilla near the end of the cooking process. Stir and serve warm or cold. Refrigerate any leftovers. *Serves 4*

Variation: Whip two free-range eggs and slowly add to the tapioca mixture while simmering. This silky pudding is a favorite of children and adults who are underweight or athletes who need to add bulk.

Gluten-free	Casein-free	Yeast-free	Soy-free	Egg-free

Trifle Bamboo Fruit Cake

Preparation Time: 30 minutes

1 Angel Food Cake (page 124)
4 cups vanilla-flavored coconut yogurt*
2 cups organic red grapes
1 cup fresh organic strawberries, cut into ¹/₄-inch slices
2 or 3 large organic bananas, cut into ¹/₄-inch slices

Cut the cake horizontally into two layers.. Place the first layer on the bottom of a trifle bowl or a cylinder-shaped glass dessert dish. Spread a 1-inch layer of the coconut yogurt on the cake. Cut the grapes into halves and arrange a layer of grapes on the side of the glass with the cut side facing out. Fill the layer with the strawberries and bananas. Repeat with the remaining cake layer, yogurt and fruit. Top with the remaining yogurt. Place one strawberry and a few grapes in the center and garnish with a mint sprig. *Serves 10 to 12*

Variation: For individual servings, cut the cake into chunks and alternate layers of cake and fresh fruit of choice in individual dessert dishes.

Note: You can make the cake the day before a party and then assemble the dessert the day of the party. Cover the top of the dish with plastic wrap to keep the cake moist.

Gluten-free	Casein-free	Egg-free	Soy-free	Yeast-free	Nut-free

Ready, Set, Eat!

Shopping Guide

Bread *(sandwich bread, tortillas, animal cookies)*
Kinnikinnick Foods, Inc.
www.kinnikinnick.com

Ener-G Foods, Inc.
www.ener-g.com

Food for Life Brown Rice Tortillas
www.organicdirect.com

Cereals *(granola, gluten-free oatmeal)*
Bakery on Main
www.bakeryonmain.com

Cream Hill Estates
www.creamhillestates.com

Glutenfreeda Foods, Inc.
www.glutenfreedafoods.com

Coconut Products *(kefir, yogurt, milk, ice cream)*
Inner-eco
www.inner-eco.com

Turtle Mountain, LLC
www.SoDeliciousDairyFree.com

Wilderness Family Naturals
www.wildernessfamilynaturals.com

Condiments *(butter substitutes, syrups, honey)*
Earth Balance *(gluten-, casein-, dairy-free, vegan margarine)* (registered trademark of GFA Brands, Inc.)
www.EarthBalanceNatural.com

Honey Gardens, Inc.
www.honeygardens.com

Wholesome Sweeteners
www.OrganicSugars.biz

Drinks *(almond, hemp, goat, raw milks)*
Blue Diamond Growers
www.almondbreeze.com

Meyenberg Goat Milk Company
www.meyenberg.com

Raw Milk
(certified un-homogenized)
www.realmilk.com

Hemp Milk
www.pacificfoods.com

Entrées *(gluten-free chicken strips, hot dogs, bacon)*
Applegate Farm
www.applegatefarms.com

Bell & Evans
www.bellandevans.com

Boar's Head Deli Meats
www.boarshead.com

Flours and Breading
Authentic Foods
www.authenticfoods.com

Bob's Red Mill Natural Foods, Inc.
www.bobsredmill.com

Honeyville Food Products
www.honeyvillegrain.com

Wilderness Family Naturals
www.wildernessfamilynaturals.com

Gluten-Free Grains, Chips, and Pasta
Ancient Harvest Quinoa
www.quinoa.net

Lundberg Family Farms
www.lundberg.com

Tinkyada
www.tinkyada.com

Nut Butters
Mara Natha Organic Nut Butters
www.maranathafoods.com

Baking Mixes *(cakes, puddings)*
Gluten-Free Pantry
www.glutino.com

Mates Vanilla Pudding Mix
www.morinu.com

Namaste Foods, LLC
www.namastefoods.com

Snacks *(crackers, cheese, pretzels, chocolate chips, bars)*
Daiya Dairy-Free Cheese
www.daiyafoods.com

Eden Organic
www.edenfoods.com

Ener-G Foods, Inc.
www.ener-g.com

Enjoy Life Natural Brands
www.enjoylife.com

Food Should Taste Good, Inc.
www.foodshouldtastegood.com

Glutino
www.glutino.com

KIND Healthy Snacks
www.kindsnacks.com

Nutiva
www.nutiva.com

Gluten-Free Soups and Stocks
Kitchen Basics Real Cooking Stocks
www.kitchenbasics.net

Gluten-Free Spices and Sugars
Penzeys Spices
(not all gluten-free)
www.penzeys.com

Wholesome Sweeteners
www.OrganicSugars.biz

Certified Gluten-Free Vanilla
www.kingarthurflour.com

Skin and Hair Care
Desert Essence
www.desertessence.com

Gluten-Free Savonnerie & Dakota Free
(mention Faye Elahi)
www.gfsoap.com, www.dakotafree.com

Testing Laboratories
Metametrix Clinical Laboratories
www.metametrix.com

Enterolab
www.enterolab.com

Gluten-Free, Allergen-Free, Toxin-Free Nutrition Supplement Manufacturers
Douglas Laboratories
www.douglaslabs.com

Klaire Labs
(a division of ProThera, Inc.)
www.klaire.com

NuMedica
www.numedica.com

Orthomolecular Products–Springboard
www.OrthoMolecularProducts.com

Speak *(fish oil supplements)*
www.SpeechNutrients.com

Organic Farms in Texas
Sand Creek Farm
(certified un-homogenized raw milk producer; between Calvert and Cameron)

North Star Ranch
(grass-fed beef, naturally raised pork, no antibiotics, no growth hormones; delivers to Dallas Farmers' Market Friday and Saturday)
www.northstarranch.net

Hiram Farm
Pat Gaines, owner
(organic greens and eggs)
Hiramfarm@sbcglobal.net

Green Gardening Tips
(For safe, green pesticide tips)
www.safelawns.com

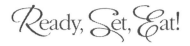

Government Research Organizations and Approved Nonprofit Listings

Government Research Organizations

Barrett's Esophagus
www.barrettsinfo.com

Centers for Disease Control and Prevention
www.cdc.gov

U.S. Food and Drug Administration
www.fda.gov

Medical Organizations and Societies

American Partnership for Eosinophilic Disorders
www.apfed.org

American Gastroenterological Association
www.gastro.org

International Foundation for Functional Gastrointestinal Disorders
www.iffgd.org

North American Society for Pediatric Gastroenterology, Hepatology, and Nutrition
www.naspghan.org

Pediatric/Adolescent Gastroesophageal Reflux Association
www.reflux.org

Society of Amercan Gastrointestinal Endoscopic Surgeons
www.sages.org

Approved Nonprofit Listings

Gluten Intolerance Group of North America
www.gluten.net
253-833-6655
info@gluten.net

University of Chicago Celiac Disease Center
www.celiacdisease.net
773-702-0666
info@celiacdisease.net

Celiac Disease Foundation
www.celiac.org
818-990-2354
cdf@celiac.org

American Celiac Disease Alliance
www.american celiac.org
703-622-3331
info@americanceliac.org

ROCK—Raising Our Celiac Kids
www.dallasrock.org
972-442-9328
leader@dallas.org

Celiac Sprue Association
www.csaceliacs.org
877-272-4272
celiacs@csaceliacs.org

Autism Society
www.autism-society.org
800-3AUTISM (800-328-8476)
info@autism-society.org

Autism Research Institute
www.autism.com
866-366-3361 parent line
619-281-7165

ADDA SR
www.adda-sr.org
281-897-0982
addaoffice@sbcglobal.net

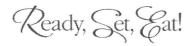

Substitutions

Instead of	Use
All-Purpose Flour (for any baked good)	Blend: 1 cup white rice flour 1/2 cup gluten-free oat flour 1/4 cup plus 2 tablespoons coconut flour Makes 2 cups
High-Protein Flour (for crusty potpie, scones)	Blend: 1 1/4 cups navy bean flour or garbanzo bean flour 1 cup arrowroot powder or potato starch 1 cup tapioca flour 1 cup brown rice flour Makes 4 1/4 cups
Self-Rising Flour (for muffins, cupcakes, cakes, or pancakes)	Blend: 1 1/4 cups white rice flour 1 1/4 cups millet flour (or sorghum flour) 1/2 cup tapioca flour 2 teaspoons xanthan gum (binding agent used for cakes, muffins, breads) 4 teaspoons gluten-free baking powder 1/2 teaspoon organic sea salt* *Note:* For a successful pizza crust, use 1 teaspoon of xanthan gum per cup of self-rising flour.
Note: Mix the above three blends using the amounts given, or double or triple the recipe and store in the refrigerator in a glass airtight container until used.	
Buttermilk	1 cup coconut milk, or 7/8 cup gluten-free plain rice milk *Note:* The above ratios are the equivalent of 1 cup buttermilk.
Egg	1 tablespoon flaxseed meal plus 3 tablespoons warm water (Let stand for 5 minutes until thickened.) 3 tablespoons no-sugar-added applesauce plus 1 teaspoon arrowroot powder *Note:* The above substitutions are the equivalent of 1 large egg. To replace an egg white, dissolve 1 tablespoon plain agar powder in 1 tablespoon water.
Yogurt	1 cup coconut yogurt (plain) 1 cup unsweetened applesauce 1 cup pear sauce *Note:* The above substitutions are the equivalent of 1 cup yogurt.
Nuts	Toasted shredded coconut Crushed toasted sunflower seeds Powdered crunchy flax cereal

Oils

Oil Type	Satu-rated	Mono-unsaturated	Poly-unsaturated	Smoke Point	Uses
Butter	66%	30%	4%	302 °F	cooking, baking, condiment, sauces, flavoring
Ghee, clarified butter	65%	32%	3%	374–482 °F	deep frying, cooking, sautéing, condiment, flavoring
Canola oil	6%	62%	32%	468 °F	frying, baking, salad dressings
Coconut oil	92%	6%	2%	351 °F	commercial baked goods, candy and sweets, whipped toppings, nondairy coffee creamers, shortening
Rice bran oil	20%	47%	33%	489 °F	cooking, frying, deep frying, salad dressings. very clean flavored and palatable
Corn oil	13%	25%	62%	457 °F	frying, baking, salad dressings, margarine, shortening
Cottonseed oil	24%	26%	50%	421 °F	margarine, shortening, salad dressings, commercially fried products
Grapeseed oil	12%	17%	71%	399 °F	cooking, salad dressings, margarine
Lard	41%	47%	33%	280–394 °F	baking, frying
Margarine, hard	80%	14%	6%	302 °F	cooking, baking, condiment
Margarine, soft	20%	47%	33%	302–320 °F	cooking, baking, condiment
Diacyl-glycerol (DAG) oil	3.5%	37.95%	59%	419 °F	frying, baking, salad oil

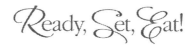

Oils

Oil Type	Satu-rated	Mono-unsaturated	Poly-unsaturated	Smoke Point	Uses
Olive oil (extra virgin)	14%	73%	11%	374 °F	cooking, salad oils, margarine (Extra light olive oil's smoke point is 468 °F)
Peanut oil	18%	49%	33%	448 °F	frying, cooking, salad oils, margarine
Safflower oil	10%	13%	77%	509 °F	cooking, salad dressings, margarine
Sesame oil (semi-refined)	14%	43%	43%	351 °F	cooking
Soybean	15%	24%	61%	466 °F	cooking, salad dressings, vegetable oil, margarine, shortening
Sunflower oil (linoleic)	11%	20%	69%	475 °F	cooking, salad dressings, margarine, shortening

General Dietary Guidelines

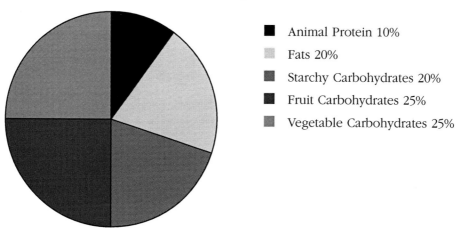

■ Animal Protein 10%

▨ Fats 20%

▨ Starchy Carbohydrates 20%

■ Fruit Carbohydrates 25%

▨ Vegetable Carbohydrates 25%

Toxic Metals

Aluminum	Antimony	Arsenic	Beryllium	Bismuth	Cadmium	Lead
tea kettles	environ-mental pollution	wood preserva-tives	high-tech consumer products	some pharma-ceuticals	shellfish	fluorescent lighting
drinking water	flame-retardant pajamas	alloying agents	gemstones	some OTC stomach remedies	some grains	drinking water
some flour tortillas	flame-retardant paint	mining, industrial mission	hardening agent in alloys		metal plates	some candy
some coffee creamers	chemical base of plastic	drinking water	planned space telescopes		plastic	paint
some dried cake, muffin & bread mixes	fireworks	picnic tables	rocket nozzles		pigment	emissions
chemical leavening agents (i.e., baking soda	alloyed with tin to make pewter itens: cups	playground equipment	filters		batteries	industrial exposures
processed food: grain, cheese, vegetables, herbs, tea	medicine	poisonous agent	windows in radiation experiments		highly toxic gas from burning oil	some toys
buffered analgesics, antacids	99.99% pure form used in semi-conductor				toxic gas from burning fossil fuel	pesticides
aluminum foil wrap						glass containers
pots & pans						cosmetics
vaccines						some tableware

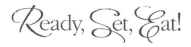

Toxic Metals*

Mercury	Nickel	Platinum	Thallium	Thorium	Tin	Tungsten
flourescent lighting	costume jewelry	old thermometers	smoking cigarettes	hazardous waste sites	pots & pans	metal-working
drinking water	eyeglass frames	jewelry	exposure to hazardous waste sites	contaminated soil & water	rubber	construction & electrical machinery
batteries	silver & white gold jewelry	containers	contaminated soils & water		plastic	Transportation equipment
fungicides	hairpins	catalyst			Alloyed with antimony for pewter	lightbulb filaments
paint	chairs					carbide in drilling equipment
disinfectants	dental braces					Heat & radiation shielding
emissions	flatware					textile dyes
amalgams	coins					enamels
industrial waste	medical instruments					glass paint
some preservatives	hair dye					
some toys	bleaching agents					
some pharmaceuticals	chemical fertilizers					
vaccines	pots & pans					
old thermometers	mineral oil products					
some fish oils	table salt					
seafood						

*Uranium: nephro-toxin

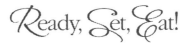

Nutrients and Symptoms Relationship Table
by Faye Elahi

Body Area	Clinical Signs/ Symptoms	Associated Nutrient(s) Deficiencies	Associated Condition
Circulation	Poor clotting	Vitamin K	
	Elevated homocysteine	Vitamin B6, methyl B12, folate	Inflammation
	Fatigue, lethargy	Iron, vitamin B12, essential fatty acid	Anemia
Digestive Tract	Belching, burping, bloating	Low stomach acid	Digestive enzyme deficiency, food intolerance
	Chronic constipation	Bacterial overgrowth, low magnesium	Gut dysbiosis, gluten intolerance
	Diarrhea	Bacterial overgrowth, low protein detoxification factor insufficiency	Heavy metal toxicity, gluten intolerance or celiac disease
	Inflamamation of colon		
	Nausea	Vitamin B6, Zinc	
Ears	Thick ear wax	Essential fatty acids (omega 3), vitamin A	Vegans, fat-, dairy-, or fish-restricted diets, autism spectrum disorders (ASD), celiac disease, food allergies, heavy metal toxicity
	Ringing in ears (tinnitus)	Niacin or B3	
	Itching	Vitamin A, zinc, yeast overgrowth	Yeast overgrowth
Eyes	Bloodshot, itchy eyes	Vitamin B2	Sjögren's disease
	Dry eyes	Essential fatty acids/ vitamin A	Food allergies, celiac disease
	Macular degeneration	Zinc, alpha lipoic acid, fatty acids	Circulatory dysfunction
	Sideways glance	Vitamin A	ASD, celiac disease, food allergies
	Sensitivity to light	Vitamin A	Sensory integration disorder (SID), ASD, celiac disease
Growth	Short stature, growth delays	Protein, zinc, vitamin A, vitamin B, calcium, essential fatty acids	Celiac disease, small intestinal malabsorption
Hair	Hair loss (alopecia)	Biotin, protein, zinc	Celiac disease & gluten sensitivity
	Dry hair, lackluster		Hypothyroidism
Head	Frontal (forehead) bulging	Calcium, vitamin D3	Autism spectrum disorder (ASD), vitamin D deficiency, celiac disease

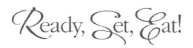

Nutrients and Symptoms Relationship Table

by Faye Elahi

Body Area	Clinical Signs/ Symptoms	Associated Nutrient(s) Deficiencies	Associated Condition
Hormones	Cold intolerance	B vitamin, essential fatty acids	Hypothyroidism, poor circulation
	Low blood sugar (hypoglycemia)	Chromium, zinc, magnesium, biotin	Insulin insufficiency, glucose intolerance, diabetes
	High blood sugar (hyperglycemia)		
	Excessive sweating	Vitamin D3, essential fatty acids	
Liver	High alkaline Phosphatase	Vitamin A or vitamin D3	Celiac disease, malabsorption, heavy metal toxicity
	Enzyme imbalance	Essential fatty acids, amino acids	
Lungs	Tightening of chest Wheezing	Essential fatty acids, vitamin D3	Asthma, food allergies, food intolerances, celiac disease, gluten sensitivity
	Shortness of breath	Vitamin D3, essential fatty acids (anti-inflammatory properties)	Anxiety, nervousness
Muscles	Bowed legs	Vitamin D3, calcium, magnesium, zinc	Poor nutrition, celiac disease, picky eating, sensory integration disorder (SID)
	Low muscle tone	Exercise core muscles, zinc, protein	Gait imbalance
Nails	White spots	Severe zinc deficiency	
	Ridges (vertical lines)	Essential fatty acids	Adrenal fatigue, anxiety
	Splitting	Protein, calcium, magnesium	Malabsorption
	Thick nails	Probiotics, antifungal	Fungus
Neuro-logical	Burning feet	Vitamin B5 (pantothenic acid)	
	Restless leg, loss of sensation in hands/feet	Essential fatty acids, vitamin E	Peripheral neuropathy, celiac disease, gluten sensitivity, malabsorption
		Magnesium methyl B12, vitamin Bs	
	Problems moving arms/legs, with balance	Vitamins B2, B6 and methyl B12, multiple vitamins and minerals	Multiple sclerosis
	Muscle spasms (startle reflex)	Mineral deficiencies: iron, zinc	
	Seizures	Multiple minerals, vitamin B6, taurine	Grand mal and petit mal seizures, quadraplegia, celiac disease
Nose	Loss of smell	Zinc	Sensory integration disorder

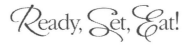

Nutrients and Symptoms Relationship Table
by Faye Elahi

Body Area	Clinical Signs/ Symptoms	Associated Nutrient(s) Deficiencies	Associated Condition
Psycho-logical	Depression, mental apathy	Severe B vitamins, essential fatty acids, magnesium	Chronic depression
	Severe mood change, aggression, euphoria	B vitamins, taurine, magnesium, vitamin E, essential fatty acids	Schizophrenia/bipolar disorder
	Food addiction, eating disorders	B vitamins, multiple minerals (zinc, magnesium, iron)	Food allergies, food intolerances
	Mental fogginess	B vitamins, multiple minerals	Celiac disease, gluten sensitivity, food allergies, malabsorption
	Eating nonfoods	Mineral deficiencies: iron, zinc, magnesium, calcium	Pica condition
Skin	Eczema, red dry patches behind neck, knees, elbows	Essential fatty acids, severe vitamin and mineral deficiencies	Dermatitis herpetiformis, celiac disease, gluten sensitivity, severe malabsorption of protein and minerals
	Acne, blemishes	Zinc	Acne, food allergies, and intolerances
	Skin peeling	Essential fatty acids, bacterial overgrowth	Fungus, vitamin A overdose (rare)
	Rough scaly skin	Essential fatty acids, vitamin D3, zinc	Celiac disease, gluten sensitivity
Urinary Tract	Urinary tract or genital itching, burning, redness, rash	Compromised immune system, yeast overgrowth, acidic system	Urinary tract infection (carbohydrate-rich diet), food allergies, candidiasis
	Kidney stones	Magnesium, calcium Vitamin B6	High oxalate diet

Sources

ADHD—A Complete Authoritative Guide, (American Academy of Pediatrics); Micheal I. Reiff, MD, FAAP, Editor-in-chief, with Sherill Tippins, AAP Publisher, 2004.

"Aluminum info: Redhead K," Quinlan GJ, Das RG, Gutteridge JM. Pharmacol Toxicol 1992 Apr; 70 (4): 278-80.

"Autistic therapies focused by Laboratory Data. Part 1. Organic Acids," Dr. Richard S. Lord, PhD, Winter 2005.

Batteries: http://www.epa.gov/hg/consumer.htm

"Breaking the Vicious Cycle: Intestinal Health through Diet," Elaine Gloria Gottschall. Kirkton Press, 1994.

Dangerous Grains, James Braly, MD, and Ron Hoggan, MA. Penguin Putnam, 2002.

"Dangers of High Fructose Corn Syrup, The," by John Mericle MD. Enzine Articles, 2005.

Devil in the Milk: Health and the Politics of A1 and A2 Milk, Keith Woodford. First Chelsea Green Printing, 2009.

"Economic benefits of increased diagnosis of celiac disease in a national managed care population in the United States," Green PH, Neugul AL, Naiyer AJ, Edwards ZC, Gabinelle S, Chinburapa V. *J Insur Med.* 2008; 40 (3-4):218-28.

Essential Gluten-Free Restaurant Guide, The, Triumph Dining Gluten-Free Publishing, 4th edition 2009.

Food and Behavior, Barbara Reed Stitts. Natural Press 2004.

Harrison's Principles of Internal Medicine, A.S. Fauci, 14th ed. New York: McGraw Hill, 1998:510, Sporn, et al. 531-532, 535.

Healing the New Childhood Epidemics: Autism, ADHD, Asthma, and Allergies, Kenneth Bock, MD and Cameron Stauth. Ballantine Books, 2008.

"Is one trans fat, CLC, better than the others?" by J. Strax, September 9, 2003. Updated and re-edited April 20, 2006. Sources: University of Iowa Health Center; Mark Moyad; PUBMED.

List of gluten foods, May 1997. Sprue-Nik News.

    (1) Federal Register (4-1-96 Edition) 21CFR Ch.1, Section 184.12277.

    (2) Federal Register (4-1-96) 21 CFR. Ch.1, Section 184.1444

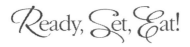

Next Green Revolution: Essential Steps to a Healthy Sustainable Agriculture, The, Raymond P. Poincelot, James E. Horne, PhD, Maura McDermott. The Haworth Press, Inc., 2001.

"Nutrition Reviews"—A review of 5 studies on vitamin D status in Canada & the U.S., Mona Calvo. Food & Drug Administration, March 2003.

Out-of-Sync Child, The, Carol Stock Kranowitz, MA. Skylight Press, 2005.

Parents, Teens, and Boundaries: How to Draw the Line, Jane Bluestein, PhD. Health Communications, Inc., 1993.

"Small Intestinal histopathology and mortality risk in celiac disease," Ludvigsson JF, Montgomery SM, Ekborn A., Brandt L., Granath F., *JAMA* 2009 Sep 16:302 (11):171-8.

"Toxicology of Aluminum in the Brain: a review," Yokel RA. Neurotoxicology. 2000 Oct: (5): 813-28.

"Vaccine," 1991 Oct; 9 (10): 699-702. Review PMID: 1759487; UI: 92101590 http://www.testfoundation.org/aluminumvaccines.htm

"Vaccines and Autism," Bernard Rimland, PhD, Woody McGinnis, MD, Autism Research Institute, San Diego, California; Published in *Laboratory Medicine*, September 2002, Issue 9, Volume 33.

"Why You Should Avoid Trans Fatty Acids," Brian Olshansky, MD. University of Iowa Health Sciences, http://www.uihealthcare.com/topics/medical departments/internalmedicine/transfattyacids/index.html, October 2003.

"Autism & Mercury: More on Mercury & Autism," Boyd D. Haley, PhD: Mercury Toxicity as it Relates to Neurological Damage in Autism Spectrum Disorders www.altcorp.com. Toxins: www.metametrix.com

Adverse reactions after injection of absorbed diptheria pertussis-tetanus (DPT) vaccine are not due only to pertussis organisms or pertussis components in the vaccine.

College of Pharmacy and Graduate Center for Toxicology, University of Kentucky Medical Center, Lexington, USA. Ryokel1@pop.uky.edu

http://www.testfoundation.org/aluminumvaccines.htm

Studies aim to resolve confusion over mercury risks from fish

Research identifies riskier fish and ways to limit potentially harmful exposures, Janet Raloff

Ready, Set, Eat!

Recipe Index

(**Bold** page numbers indicate photo recipes.)

Ready, Set, Eat!

User Guide Index

About the Author

Faye Elahi, MS, MA, practices Orthomolecular Nutrition, which gives the body what it needs in safe amounts. Drawing from her psychology and nutrition background, Faye uses dietary and nutrition therapies to address emotional, behavioral, and nutritional imbalances. These nonintrusive therapies are inexpensive and safe, with proven results.

Her research work has been published in the professional *Journal of The American Dietetic Association*. Faye's areas of specialty are celiac disease, autism spectrum disorder, Asperger's syndrome, attention deficit disorder, Down syndrome, and diabetes. Currently she serves as a nutrition advisor for the DFW Lone Star Celiac Support Group and several physician groups in the Dallas Metroplex.

Faye holds masters degrees in nutrition, child psychology, and mass communications. Since 1998, she has worked with patients at her nutrition practice in the North Dallas area. She is married and has two children.

To order additional copies of Faye's book, *Ready, Set, Eat!*, please visit her Web site: www.glutenfreenutritionforlife.com.